Running

The Inspirational Journey of a Non-runner

(The Ultimate Runner's Guide to Make You Healthy, Ignite Your Run, and Embrace Wellness)

Harry Duke

Published By **Frank Joseph**

Harry Duke

All Rights Reserved

Running: The Inspirational Journey of a Non-runner (The Ultimate Runner's Guide to Make You Healthy, Ignite Your Run, and Embrace Wellness)

ISBN   978-1-7774070-1-8

Legal & Disclaimer

Table Of Contents

Chapter 1: Fundamentals Of Endurance Training

1.1 ENERGY SYSTEMS

This phase of the e-book on electricity structures is vital for statistics the inner workings of the human body, how energy is generated, and the importance of electricity manufacturing.

All the dwelling tissues in our our our bodies continuously call for strength to function optimally. This energy is derived from the synthesis of Adenosine Triphosphate (ATP), an strength-wearing molecule often called the "power distant places money of life" or the "fuel of life." ATP serves due to the fact the general power supply for all living cells, making it the cornerstone of strength manufacturing. Every residing organism, which include ourselves, includes cells that depend on ATP to fulfill their energy necessities. Without ATP, cells ought to lack the gas and energy vital for wearing out critical capabilities, ultimately critical to their dying. Thus, ATP is critical for the survival and functioning of all styles of existence.

Muscles, being dwelling tissues much like the relaxation of our body, rely on ATP to execute a tremendous sort of functions, from normal sports like walking and going for walks to greater intense actions which includes leaping and sprinting.

The food we consume undergoes a chain of chemical reactions that smash it down into ATP, permitting the severa features of our body, along side muscle feature. This device, which involves transforming the nutrients from our healthy eating plan into ATP molecules that offer the crucial strength required by using our muscle tissue, constitutes the essence of electricity production.

Our frame makes use of 3 considered considered one of a kind strength structures from which ATP production takes vicinity: the aerobic electricity tool, the anaerobic-lactic energy machine, and the anaerobic-alactic power system.

The cardio energy machine produces ATP inside the presence of oxygen, even as the two anaerobic systems feature without oxygen. Both cardio and anaerobic metabolisms offer the crucial ATP for the body to feature in taken into consideration considered one of a type conditions. It is vital to phrase that there may be continually a aggregate of cardio and anaerobic electricity manufacturing, and there isn't always a surprising switch that changes the power manufacturing from definitely aerobic to virtually anaerobic. You'll rapid understand this idea and see how topics honestly paintings.

The fewer chemical steps an power system has to generate ATP, the more suddenly ATP is produced. This speedy production of energy permits your muscle mass to generate fast and explosive movements. However, the downside is that this electricity does no longer very last long in advance than fatigue gadgets in. This principle applies to the two anaerobic electricity systems. On the alternative hand, the cardio strength machine relies on more complex chemical reactions, due to this it takes longer to generate ATP. However, as a give up end result, greater ATP molecules are produced, bearing in mind sustained strength and electricity output over an extended time body, in spite of the truth that not as powerfully as the 2 anaerobic systems.

THE ANAEROBIC-ALACTIC ENERGY SYSTEM

The anaerobic alactic strength machine, moreover referred to as the ATP-PC (Adenosine Triphosphate-Phosphocreatine) machine, is capable of generating the quickest and most powerful muscle moves. This system has the fewest chemical reactions the various three structures, which contributes to its tempo and strength. The alactic tool does now not rely upon oxygen and does not damage down the food we eat, in comparison to the alternative energy structures, to deliver ATP. Instead, it is predicated on small amounts of ATP and phosphocreatine saved inside the muscle tissue.

However, the very limited quantity of stored ATP and phosphocreatine within the muscle agencies can only offer strength for round 10 seconds. After this time frame, the alactic system is not capable of supply strength because it depletes its stored muscle reserves (ATP and PC). During the number one 2 seconds of intense exercising at maximum effort, strength needs are met through the stored ATP. After 2 seconds, ATP is depleted, and muscle phosphocreatine lets in regenerate ATP for a few other 8 seconds of most depth exercising.

It is crucial to observe that the alactic machine "runs out of gasoline" inside those 10 seconds while exerting a hundred% intensity. However, at submaximal ranges, the device can generate electricity for a barely longer length. Understanding this is crucial due to the fact, for instance, going for walks at eighty 5% of top pace for 10 seconds will take a bit greater time for the alactic tool to expend its stored reserves.

Additionally, the aerobic system is responsible for replenishing the constructing blocks and enzymes required with the resource of the use of the alactic machine to generate ATP as soon because it runs out of its reserves. The higher advanced one's aerobic tool is, the faster the alactic device will recover. Generally, if whole healing is authorized amongst maximal alactic efforts, it takes approximately 30 seconds to replenish about 70% of the phosphocreatine and approximately three to 5 minutes to top off 100%. A nicely-superior aerobic device permits quicker restoration of the alactic tool.

In phrases of development capability, the alactic device has confined room for improvement, with genetic effect gambling a terrific feature. Among the three power systems, it gives the least possibility for improvement.

THE ANAEROBIC-LACTIC ENERGY SYSTEM

The anaerobic-lactic or glycolytic gadget is the alternative anaerobic device that does not rely upon oxygen for ATP production. However, the essential component distinction among the lactic gadget and the alactic machine is that the lactic gadget does no longer hire saved PC (phosphocreatine) from the muscle organizations for strength manufacturing. Instead, it's far predicated at the breakdown of carbohydrates to generate ATP.

During anaerobic glycolysis, carbohydrates in the shape of every blood sugar (glucose) or saved sugar (glycogen) damage down thru a sequence of chemical reactions to form pyruvate without the usage of oxygen. When glycogen is broken down into glucose, it is called glycogenolysis.

For each molecule of glucose damaged right the entire manner all the way down to pyruvate, molecules of ATP are produced, which may be utilized by the strolling muscle tissue.

GLYCOLYSIS

Once pyruvate is shaped, matters can occur. It can be converted proper right into a molecule called Acetyl CoA, which enters the mitochondria and, via a series of chemical steps and with the presence of oxygen, generates 32 ATP molecules. This pathway of electricity manufacturing is aerobic. While the method begins offevolved offevolved anaerobically without the presence of oxygen, cardio power manufacturing takes place while pyruvate will become Acetyl CoA and enters the mitochondria. This method is called cardio glycolysis.

The specific opportunity is the conversion of pyruvate into lactate. For every lactate molecule produced, one hydrogen ion (H+) is likewise commonplace. This technique is the anaerobic lactic or glycolytic electricity manufacturing, and it produces 2 ATP molecules in line with glucose molecule. The production of lactate is the purpose this device is known as anaerobic lactic. In assessment, in alactic strength manufacturing, no lactate is produced, subsequently it's far known as alactic.

At this point, it's miles important to phrase that lactate and hydrogen ions are not absolutely produced at the identical time as there may be an inadequate amount of oxygen to satisfy the muscle's wishes. In truth, lactate is produced even at low intensities of workout or maybe at relaxation, wherein there can be an abundance of oxygen available.

While lactate and hydrogen ions are produced at each excessive and espresso intensities, there's a great distinction in their future depending on the schooling depth. When there's sufficient oxygen present, together with sooner or later of rest or low-intensity exercising, the lactate produced may be transformed lower back into pyruvate and enter the cardio metabolism pathways, at the equal time as hydrogen ions are carried away. In the diagram above, you can have a look at the arrows from pyruvate to lactate and from lactate lower back to pyruvate. Subsequently, pyruvate is converted to Acetyl CoA, and aerobic metabolism takes area. In the ones conditions, there's a balance amongst lactate manufacturing and elimination. Lactate is produced anaerobically, however its elimination happens manner to enough oxygen and aerobic metabolism. This technique maintains till the anaerobic threshold is reached. The anaerobic threshold is the maximum workout depth at which the charge of lactate production equals the fee of lactate elimination. This manner that at the same time as lactate degrees are prolonged in evaluation to resting tiers, the attention of lactate stays stable and does now not growth through the years due to the balanced expenses of producing and clearance/removal.

However, at intensities above the anaerobic threshold, there may be a unexpected increase in lactate and hydrogen ions in evaluation to intensities under the anaerobic threshold. At this thing, the rate of lactate manufacturing exceeds the rate of lactate clearance, predominant to the accumulation of lactate and hydrogen ions over time and resulting in volatile lactate levels.

It is vital to phrase that the burning sensation in muscle tissue during excessive-intensity workout routines above the lactate threshold isn't always due to lactate itself. This notion is antique, and the parable has been debunked. The actual motive of this sensation is the accumulation of hydrogen ions that can't be certainly cleared, as their manufacturing exceeds the elimination price beyond this diploma of exercising depth, as I stated earlier. These acidic ions, in choice to lactate, decrease the pH of the mobile and intrude with muscular contraction. In less complicated terms, it isn't lactate that reasons fatigue however the hydrogen ions produced simultaneously with lactate. In truth, some scientists now believe that the manufacturing of lactate truely facilitates muscle mass dispose of fatigue inside the direction of intense workout. However, despite the fact that lactate accumulation does not straight away reason fatigue and the burning sensation sooner or later of exercise, higher lactate stages can feature a reliable indicator of multiplied hydrogen ion tiers and, therefore, a extra nation of fatigue.

Furthermore, there was a protracted-fame notion that lactate is liable for the muscle discomfort expert with the aid of the usage of individuals the day after exercising. However, this belief has been examined to be totally wrong. Muscle pain that takes location post-workout is genuinely because of micro-tears and harm to the muscle fibers incurred at some stage in education. With sufficient rest and recovery, muscle ache subsides. It's essential to be conscious that lactate does now not linger in the muscle groups the day after a exercise and is typically cleared internal an hour after workout.

So, while we analyzed how glycolysis works, we can classify it into instructions: cardio glycolysis and anaerobic glycolysis. The preliminary phase of the method constantly happens inside the absence of oxygen, however the ensuing very last outcomes varies based totally completely mostly on whether or not or now not pyruvate is converted into Acetyl CoA (aerobic glycolysis) or lactate (anaerobic glycolysis). It's vital to be aware that even in the course of low-depth exercising, anaerobic glycolysis continues to be gift. However, at intensities beneath the anaerobic threshold, lactate can convert again to pyruvate and enter cardio metabolism. As exercise intensity surpasses the anaerobic threshold, anaerobic glycolysis will become greater fantastic.

In regard to the power production of anaerobic glycolysis, this device is capable of a higher price of ATP manufacturing in comparison to the aerobic gadget, however decrease than the alactic device. It falls amongst these structures in terms of the price of ATP production.

When it involves the duration of strength manufacturing through anaerobic lactic metabolism, it normally lasts round forty seconds whilst the depth is at most attempt. As we determined with alactic metabolism, which depletes its energy shops inside 10 seconds at maximum depth but can be sustained for a piece longer at submaximal intensities, a comparable precept applies right here. If the exercising depth is decrease than this, which can be sustained for about forty seconds, anaerobic lactic electricity manufacturing can hold for a chunk greater than forty seconds. However, all through any excessive-depth strive, past about fifty 5 to 60 seconds, cardio metabolism considerably contributes to energy manufacturing.

Concerning the ability for improvement in this device, the reality is that at the same time as it could be advanced barely extra than the alactic gadget, it does not have a massive ceiling. Training diversifications that occur with this type of education may be maximized in four-6 weeks.

Chapter 2: The Aerobic Energy System

The aerobic electricity machine uses oxygen to supply ATP, in assessment to the 2 anaerobic energy systems which do no longer depend on oxygen. Additionally, it's far the first-rate power system that might destroy down both fats and carbohydrates for strength manufacturing. While the aerobic tool is capable of generating electricity for a protracted length without fatigue, it does not produce as loads energy as the 2 anaerobic structures. This extended energy production is a result of the higher ATP manufacturing of aerobic metabolism as compared to the two anaerobic structures. However, because of the complexity of the cardio metabolism and the more massive sort of chemical reactions concerned in ATP production in comparison to the alactic and glycolytic anaerobic systems, the fee of strength output is lower.

Aerobic metabolism completely takes place within the mitochondria and continually requires the presence of oxygen. There are techniques that ATP can be produced aerobically: through carbohydrate breakdown (cardio glycolysis) or fats breakdown (cardio lipolysis).

Earlier, we said the manner of aerobic glycolysis, in which pyruvate, formed from glucose, converts to Acetyl CoA and enters the mitochondria. In the presence of oxygen, severa complicated chemical steps arise, ensuing in the manufacturing of 32 ATP molecules in step with glucose molecule. In evaluation, cardio lipolysis includes using fats saved as triglycerides in adipose tissue and skeletal muscles. During cardio electricity production the use of fat, triglycerides are to start with damaged down into free fatty acids and glycerol. The unfastened fatty acids are then transported to the muscle mitochondria, in which Acetyl CoA is fashioned. Following Acetyl CoA formation, fat metabolism proceeds identically to carbohydrate metabolism. The key difference, however, lies in the quantity of strength produced. Aerobic lipolysis yields considerably greater ATP molecules in evaluation to aerobic glycolysis. While cardio glycolysis produces about 32 ATP molecules steady with glucose molecule, aerobic lipolysis can generate a mean internet of 106 ATP molecules in step with molecule of fats. It's essential to word that at the identical time as aerobic lipolysis produces greater ATP and gives longer-lasting electricity, the manner itself is slower in comparison to aerobic glycolysis. Consequently, the energy output executed thru aerobic lipolysis is decrease than that of aerobic glycolysis.

Think of the strength systems as a continuum, wherein cardio lipolysis is at the left component and anaerobic alactic is on the proper side. Aerobic glycolysis is next to aerobic lipolysis, and anaerobic glycolysis "sits" to the right aspect within the lower back of anaerobic alactic and within the the the front of aerobic glycolysis (Aerobic lipolysis - Aerobic glycolysis - Anaerobic glycolysis - Anaerobic alactic). The further an strength gadget is to the right factor, the more strength it possesses but with less functionality. Conversely, while an electricity device is within the direction of the left element, it has a whole lot a great deal less power but greater staying electricity and capability.

As referred to earlier, the alactic tool can produce strength for about 10 seconds at most intensities, at the identical time because the lactic tool can maintain energy manufacturing for about forty seconds. In regard to aerobic energy production, cardio glycolysis allows you to art work at a better strength output compared to cardio lipolysis, however now not for as long as cardio lipolysis. On the opportunity hand, fat breakdown from cardio lipolysis offers long-lasting energy, even though it generates the least electricity at the same time as in comparison to the two anaerobic structures and cardio glycolysis.

At this issue, it's far essential to keep in mind that there is always a combination of cardio glycolysis and cardio lipolysis contributing to energy production. At very low training intensities and at some stage in rest, the bulk of burned power come from fats, however carbohydrates moreover contribute to power manufacturing. As depth will boom, aerobic glycolysis becomes extra splendid, however this doesn't suggest that aerobic lipolysis stops. There is constantly a aggregate of fats and carbohydrates breaking down, as said formerly.

While the two structures of aerobic strength manufacturing usually work together, and the percentage of exertions for every one is based totally upon at the intensity and period of exercising, aerobic lipolysis can be the largest supply of strength in instances in which glycogen stores have been depleted. Glycogen is stored within the muscle companies and liver. Approximately 4 hundred grams of glycogen are saved in the muscle organizations, and spherical a hundred-a hundred twenty grams are saved in the liver. With schooling, muscle glycogen can be extended barely, however liver glycogen can't. Muscle glycogen serves as a gas supply in your muscle groups, whilst liver glycogen is accountable for regulating blood glucose levels. Additionally, blood glucose is the maximum essential supply of strength to your brain, every at rest and all through exercising.

During exercise, muscular tissues make use of their non-public glycogen shops. However, as muscle glycogen reserves usually decrease, blood glucose assumes an an increasing number of large characteristic in assembly the body's electricity wishes. When muscle glycogen is depleted, the frame is based on liver glycogen as a source of glucose to meet the muscle mass' name for. However, it's far simplest a rely of time earlier than liver glycogen stores additionally come to be all of sudden depleted. When this occurs, blood glucose tiers drop too low, fundamental to hypoglycemia, which can also moreover bring about symptoms together with complications, fatigue, and nausea. At this component, slowing down appreciably turns into the simplest viable opportunity.

In this sort of case, the frame's best alternative is to rely on fat to maintain workout. However, in spite of the truth that the majority of energy comes from fat breakdown at this factor, the frame will though produce a few glycogen from fats and proteins to hold blood glucose ranges as soon as glycogen is depleted. This device is referred to as gluconeogenesis. However, it's far crucial to look at that gluconeogenesis is not a quick or green technique, and you cannot rely on it to hold the identical degree of velocity or typical overall performance as in advance than glycogen depletion happened. Its primary position is to assist in preserving blood glucose levels after glycogen has been depleted.

The glycogen that may be crafted from fat is in negligible portions. As defined earlier in the assessment of cardio lipolysis, triglycerides are damaged down into loose fatty acids and glycerol. Free fatty acids make a contribution to energy manufacturing thru cardio lipolysis. On the alternative hand, glycerol derived from triglycerides may be transformed into glucose. However, it is crucial to phrase that glycerol represents handiest a small fraction of the fat molecule, as the majority of the triglyceride's mass includes fatty acids. Consequently, the glucose normal from glycerol is produced in minimal quantities and is inadequate to provide huge strength.

In addition to fat, glycogen additionally may be created from amino acids, which can be the building blocks of protein. If someone does not consume enough protein in line with his/her frame's goals, amino acids from the muscle tissues may be applied for glycogen synthesis. This way that the body breaks down muscle tissue to keep blood glucose inner the appropriate variety.

So, while glycogen depletion takes location, reliance on cardio lipolysis for electricity production will increase, however it comes with the disadvantage of a slower strolling pace. Energy generation from the cardio lipolytic pathway is not as inexperienced for strolling at high speeds in assessment to the aerobic glycolytic pathway, as we've were given have been given visible. However, in concept, you may keep prolonged workout using strength derived from fat breakdown. It is essential to be aware, even though, that extraordinary factors which encompass dehydration, muscular fatigue, and diverse barriers may also moreover ultimately avert your ability to hold exercise, irrespective of the capability for limitless power from aerobic lipolysis.

Speaking of countless strength, permit's bear in mind the strength capability of glycogen reserves. When glycogen reserves are whole, they are able to provide spherical 2000 energy of electricity. This calculation is primarily based on the fact that 1 gram of carbohydrates, which may be damaged down into glucose, gives four power. If we multiply the about 500 grams of popular stored glycogen within the muscle agencies and liver, it quantities to 2000 electricity. However, 2000 power can not preserve extended staying energy activities indefinitely.

In assessment to the restricted glycogen shops, body fat can offer electricity for a far longer duration. Fat is the most focused deliver of energy, offering greater than times the electricity of carbohydrates or protein. While proteins and carbohydrates yield 4 electricity in keeping with gram, fats gives nine strength regular with gram. In people with everyday weight, body fats can offer more or a good deal less forty,000-one hundred,000 electricity, counting on the quantity of fat present. In overweight humans, this amount may be even higher. Forty,000-100,000 energy represents a exquisite amount of energy.

On commonplace, the kind of power burned within the course of a marathon is round 2,six hundred. However, this discern varies from man or woman to man or woman, as people with better frame weight have a propensity to burn extra energy compared to lighter human beings. Nevertheless, 2,six hundred serves as an cheap common estimate.

Now, permit's maintain in mind how a remarkable deal power can be constituted of a hundred,000 energy, due to the fact that a median marathon requires approximately 2,600 strength. This is the purpose why, in idea, you can maintain themselves for an prolonged term completely on strength derived from fat, assuming we exclude other elements along with dehydration, muscular fatigue, and intellectual fatigue from the equation.

Regarding the time at which glycogen depletion takes place, it relies upon on every the depth and period of workout.

Assuming your glycogen shops are entire, in case you're going to run on the fastest velocity you could maintain for two hours, your glycogen will likely be depleted someplace within this time period. It's crucial to have a take a look at, but, that the two-hour mark refers specifically to the fastest tempo for this era. Many human beings misunderstand this "2-hour rule" and expect that any pace all through this time period depletes glycogen shops. If you run for 2 hours however maintain a tempo that you may keep for four hours, then your glycogen shops will now not be in reality emptied after 2 hours however as an opportunity near to 3 or three and a 1/2 of hours. Some runners recall that they deplete their glycogen shops inside the path of a protracted, smooth run lasting round ninety-100 and twenty mins at a pace they could keep for three-4 hours, however it's far now not the case. While a massive amount of stored glycogen might be used, it's far doubtful that it is going to be truly depleted. The lower the taking walks depth, the less glycogen is ate up in step with minute.

Generally, at the identical time as intensity is a huge aspect in how speedy glycogen is utilized by the frame, it takes a large amount of time for depletion to stand up. For example, taking walks at the anaerobic threshold level for an hour, that is the maximum period you can maintain this attempt, will make use of a great amount of glycogen but it won't be simply depleted. On the opportunity hand, the 2-hour maximum running pace, irrespective of being of lower intensity than the 1-hour anaerobic threshold run, permits for sufficient time to dissipate glycogen because of the 1-hour difference in duration among the 2 efforts. The identical principle applies to intensities above the anaerobic threshold. Glycogen utilization will boom unexpectedly beyond this component, however strolling at most paces above the anaerobic threshold for 40, 30, 20, or maybe 10 mins will not expend glycogen. Despite the high depth, the length is not prolonged sufficient in your muscles to exhaust their glycogen reserves.

After this thorough assessment of the aerobic power device, it's miles critical to emphasize that this energy tool offers the satisfactory capability for improvement among all of the energy systems. In reality, it takes years of education to achieve its most improvement.

Chapter 3: Energy Systems In Practice

Having analyzed every electricity system, allow's now have a look at how they feature in exercising. But earlier than we hold, it is important to understand a few schooling terms together with VO2 max, aerobic threshold, and anaerobic threshold.

In the case of uninformed trainees, there has a tendency to be huge confusion surrounding those thresholds. While the anaerobic threshold is the more normally diagnosed threshold, it's far crucial to apprehend that there is moreover an cardio threshold. It's vital to distinguish most of the 2 to avoid mixing them up, which regularly happens.

The cardio threshold is the intensity at which lactate starts to accumulate above resting tiers. As we stated in advance inside the context of strength systems, lactate is produced even at relaxation. At intensities beneath the aerobic threshold, lactate degrees stay similar to resting stages. The intensity on the aerobic threshold is considered easy, and it is sustainable for numerous hours, generally round four hours.

The aerobic threshold is often called LT1 (lactate threshold 1) or VT1 (ventilatory threshold 1). It is known as LT1 because of the increase in lactate degrees above resting levels. Resting lactate levels normally range from 0.Five to 1.Five mmol/L, with an average of round 1.Three mmol/L, however man or woman variations may additionally moreover exist. The lactate attention on the aerobic threshold is ready 2 mmol/L, although this may additionally variety amongst people. Endurance-skilled humans usually have lower lactate degrees in comparison to untrained human beings.

It additionally may be referred to as VT1 (ventilatory threshold 1) as it represents the element at which respiration price starts offevolved to growth above regular. At this intensity, breathing becomes increased but remains slight and snug, and also you enjoy capable of keeping the tempo for a extended period.

There is ongoing debate and differing evaluations concerning the relationship amongst VT1 (ventilatory threshold 1) and LT1 (lactate threshold 1), and whether they're exactly the identical. This confusion may additionally additionally rise up because of the reality some humans strictly accomplice the aerobic threshold with the appropriate lactate fee of mmol/L. However, as stated in advance, lactate values on the aerobic threshold can range amongst knowledgeable people and may be decrease than 2 mmol/L, even though they'll be actually better than resting degrees.

For instance, if an athlete's aerobic threshold is decided to be at 1.6 mmol/L of lactate, it commonly coincides with the superiority of VT1. This is due to the truth whilst lactate ranges rise above resting levels, breathing moreover starts offevolved to boom barely above everyday. However, in case you look at the precise 2 mmol/L lactate fee with the VT1 of this athlete, you'll examine that they are not exactly on the equal training intensity. The 2 mmol/L lactate rate corresponds to a barely higher depth. This is why a few argue that LT1 and VT1 aren't identical, as they strictly correlate the 2 mmol/L lactate charge with the aerobic threshold, as cited formerly.

To avoid getting misplaced in information and to simplify subjects, it may be said that the aerobic threshold, LT1, and VT1 are essentially referring to the identical point in training. This is whilst each breathing charge and lactate values are above ordinary tiers. For a few humans, lactate also can attain 2 mmol/L, at the same time as for others, it could be slightly lower.

Regarding the coronary heart rate on the cardio threshold, LT1, or VT1, it generally falls inside the sort of 75% to 79% of maximum coronary heart fee. Well-knowledgeable people will be predisposed to have coronary coronary heart expenses in the direction of 79%, on the identical time as beginners can also fall spherical seventy five% or barely decrease. When you are taking walks and function a coronary heart fee display display, paying attention to your respiratory can provide an instance of whether or not or now not you're drawing close to the aerobic threshold. You will look at that your respiration starts to upward push above normal stages, and at that element, your coronary coronary heart rate want to be inside the aforementioned range.

It's without a doubt well well worth noting that there can be a few wrong records at the internet suggesting that the coronary coronary heart fee on the aerobic threshold want to be round sixty 5% to 70% of most. However, this is not correct. Heart costs beneath 70% of most aren't in the intensity kind of the aerobic threshold. Training underneath this coronary coronary heart charge range is more suitable for recuperation skills. To confirm the depth of the aerobic threshold, it's far truly beneficial to display coronary coronary heart price or respiratory styles for the duration of workout.

The different well-known threshold is the anaerobic threshold. The anaerobic threshold is the most exercising intensity at which the fee of lactate production is equal to the charge of lactate removal, resulting in solid lactate values at this intensity. As noted within the evaluation of the anaerobic lactic power device, at intensities above the anaerobic threshold, lactate is produced at a quicker price than it may be eliminated. This outcomes in the accumulation of lactate and hydrogen ions over time, with hydrogen ions being answerable for the burning sensation and fatigue (no longer lactate itself).

Similar to the only of a type names used for the aerobic threshold, the anaerobic threshold is likewise referred to as LT2 (lactate threshold 2) or VT2 (ventilatory threshold 2).

At LT1, there can be a vital rise in lactate tiers above resting levels. Between LT1 and LT2, there can be a linear increase in lactate as the exercise depth will boom. However, internal every workout intensity variety among those elements, lactate values continue to be sturdy and do now not increase over time because of the balanced fees of lactate manufacturing and clearance. Above LT2, there may be a quick boom and accumulation of lactate because of the fee of production exceeding the rate of clearance.

It is actually simply well worth mentioning that many people often partner LT2 with a tough and fast lactate price of four mmol/L. However, much like the cardio threshold, the usage of a difficult and speedy lactate rate as a threshold length is extra of a generalization in choice to a unique fee. Well-professional staying power athletes normally exhibit lactate values amongst 3 to 3.Five mmol/L, or possibly lower, at the anaerobic threshold. On the alternative hand, folks that are lots less educated in terms of endurance or untrained humans can also moreover have lactate values at the anaerobic threshold above four mmol/L, ranging within the course of 4.Five to five mmol/L.

The concept of VT2 is similar to LT2, but in place of focusing at the upward thrust of lactate, we do not forget breathing fees. At VT1, your breathing fee will boom above everyday levels. Between

VT1 and VT2, there can be a linear growth in air drift, much like the pattern discovered with lactate ranges the various ones intensities. When strolling on the cardio threshold (VT1), you could experience which you are breathing heavier than normal, but the strive but feels feasible and relatively smooth. As the intensity will growth above VT1, respiratory continues to growth, but it stays possible. When you reach VT2, the respiratory will become particularly heavier in assessment to an awful lot a good deal much less severe efforts. However, even at this issue, it's far however a without difficulty hard effort, and you could manage it with out being certainly crushed. You have a revel in of exertion however are though capable of preserve. Above the VT2 component, the respiration charge will increase dramatically in comparison to VT2 and the intensities under it. You can without a doubt feel the distinction on the identical time as this shift occurs, due to the fact the respiration will become more tough and demanding.

So, the anaerobic threshold, LT2, or VT2 are basically the equal detail. And what applies to the aerobic threshold moreover applies right proper here. We need to now not strictly accomplice the two thresholds with the two and four mmol/L lactate values. These intensities are extra of an try-based idea, and if you are in track collectively together with your body sooner or later of your runs, it's miles fairly smooth to find out in which the thresholds are.

Regarding the strolling tempo at which the anaerobic threshold occurs, it represents the most strolling try or pace that you can preserve for 1 hour. The coronary coronary heart charge that corresponds to this attempt usually falls in the form of 88% to ninety two% of your most heart rate. For untrained humans, it could be closer to 80 5%, but with right education, it has a unethical to growth to someplace inside the 88% to ninety % variety.

The final education time period I'd like to deal with in advance than we discover how energy structures paintings in exercising is VO2 max. VO2 max represents the most amount of oxygen your body can intake and employ in step with minute, making it a diploma of your most aerobic ability. Accurate length of VO2 max calls for a ventilatory take a look at. However, even without a ventilatory lab test, it's far nonetheless possible to find out the strolling speeds related to VO2 max.

The on foot tempo that corresponds to VO2 max is an all-out try of 8 mins, it truly is a strolling velocity well above your anaerobic threshold. During the number one 1.Five-2 minutes, you are underneath one hundred% of your VO2 max as it takes about that an awful lot time to obtain one hundred% VO2 max from a standstill start at the same time as going for walks at this speed. However, after that initial duration, you're taking walks with the maximum quantity of oxygen that your body can intake and make use of. It's a really traumatic try that can't be sustained for plenty longer than this time frame.

Furthermore, many of the anaerobic threshold and VO2 max speeds, there are unique strolling paces to undergo in mind. These paces fall a few of the thresholds, being faster than the anaerobic threshold but slower than the

VO2 max pace. For instance, the most tempo you may preserve for round half of of-hour corresponds to approximately ninety% of your VO2 max. Additionally, the maximum attempt for 15 mins aligns with extra or less 90 five% of your VO2 max.

The coronary coronary heart fees associated with those efforts above the anaerobic threshold surpass 90 -ninety three% of the maximum coronary heart fee. During the 8-minute maximum try, the coronary coronary coronary heart price will probably method its maximum after the preliminary quick time. In evaluation, at some degree inside the most 30-minute pace, the coronary coronary heart charge has a bent to range spherical 94% of its most potential. The 15-minute all-out try falls somewhere within the middle, in phrases of coronary heart price, among those intensities.

It's important to be conscious that the probabilities of VO2 max related to every going for walks effort do no longer proper now correspond to the identical possibilities of the maximum heart rate that a runner reviews inside the direction of these efforts. This difference is critical to maintain in thoughts, as it's miles a commonplace deliver of misunderstanding. While 100% of VO2 max corresponds to the maximum coronary heart charge, at special opportunities of VO2 max, the percentages of most coronary coronary heart charge and VO2 max do no longer align.

For instance, 90 five% of VO2max is equivalent to ninety eight% of most coronary coronary coronary heart rate, and at ninety% of VO2max, a coronary heart price of 94% - ninety five% of the maximum is located. The coronary coronary heart price at the anaerobic threshold, which falls inside the form of 88% - ninety two% of the maximum, occurs at 80% - eighty five% of VO2max. Below the anaerobic threshold, for a most pace that you may maintain for two hours, your coronary coronary coronary heart rate may be round eighty % - 86%, in all likelihood slightly better, which corresponds to about 70% - 75% of VO2max. As we lower the intensity in addition, which consist of at some degree within the maximum pace for four hours, which represents the aerobic threshold, coronary coronary heart expenses among 75% - 79% of the maximum are decided, resulting in a far wider hole a number of the two opportunities. The coronary heart price form of seventy five% - 79% of the maximum is set 60% - 65% of VO2max. Essentially, the gap amongst coronary coronary coronary heart price and VO2max opportunities is giant at low intensities, but as intensity increases, the distance often diminishes till it reaches one hundred% VO2max, which corresponds to the maximum coronary coronary heart charge. You can see this inside the table under.

Let's move on now and find out how electricity systems characteristic at some point of numerous education intensities. First, test the subsequent photograph, which illustrates the two thresholds. It will beneficial useful resource in higher records the ideas I will talk next.

As depicted in the photo above, the 2 thresholds mark the separation of 3 education zones. While a bigger variety of zones can be useful for organizing training successfully (which I will communicate later), those three zones are enough for information how energy structures function in exercise. To beautify comprehension, it is probably beneficial to embody a in addition mark for VO2 max, placed somewhere inside the center of region 3. So, to higher draw close to the following descriptions, envision region 1 beginning with an intensity of 0 or rest, the LT1 and LT2 factors final as they are, and an imaginary line drawn in the middle of place 3 to symbolize a hundred% of VO2 max intensity.

From relaxation to the LT2 factor, the aerobic power machine gives all of the energy that your body goals. Technically, there can be anaerobic metabolism too, from relaxation to the LT2 mark because of the truth lactate is produced every at relaxation and at some stage in all intensities amongst relaxation and LT2. As we apprehend, lactate does not want the presence of oxygen to be produced. However, even as lactate is produced below LT2, it converts lower back to pyruvate after which to Acetyl CoA for cardio electricity production. Therefore, regardless of the fact that lactate manufacturing takes region, the final cease end result is its participation in aerobic energy manufacturing via reconversion. This takes region because of the equal rates of lactate manufacturing and clearance said in advance. The lactate that is produced is eliminated and takes issue in cardio metabolism. While some overly analytical "technology coaches" may additionally argue and endorse that anaerobic power production takes place underneath LT2, that is theoretically proper as I noted above, the last and full-size final results is ATP manufacturing via cardio metabolism. Hence, for simplicity and in phrases of training company, I have to say that some thing at or beneath LT2 is aerobic.

The substantial difference in how the aerobic power system operates from rest to LT2 is the ratio of fat and carbohydrate breakdown, specially aerobic lipolysis and aerobic glycolysis. Between rest and LT2 intensities, there can be constantly a mixture of fat and carbohydrate breakdown, and electricity production does no longer absolutely depend upon one or the alternative, besides in instances wherein glycogen depletion has happened. Even in the ones times, gluconeogenesis takes place via the breakdown of protein and fats. The decrease the depth, the higher the percentage of fat burned for energy, and because the intensity will boom, aerobic glycolysis will become the essential supply of energy manufacturing. While the ratios of fats and carbohydrate breakdown may additionally variety barely amongst individuals, proper right here are a few first rate not unusual possibilities:

During relaxation, spherical 80 5% of the strength produced comes from fat, while the very last 15% is derived from carbohydrates. As workout begins offevolved, the percentage of power derived from fats decreases, and the use of carbohydrates will increase. With developing depth, there may be a upward thrust in aerobic glycolysis found with the useful aid of a lower in aerobic lipolysis. At about sixty five% of VO2 max, there's an identical contribution from cardio lipolysis and aerobic glycolysis. This 50%-50% energy production ratio is normally located across the LT1 for optimum people, as the sixty five% VO2 max aligns with the coronary heart charge at the aerobic threshold. As depth further will increase beyond the LT1, the majority of energy is derived from aerobic glycolysis. At the LT2 difficulty, the power breakdown includes approximately eighty% aerobic glycolysis and 20% cardio lipolysis.

Something crucial to maintain in thoughts is that the probabilities stated above constitute the distribution of power burned. While about eighty five% of energy burned at rest come from fat, the actual sort of power burned in line with minute for the duration of rest is substantially decrease in evaluation to on foot. Similarly, the electricity burned at an intensity under the LT1 are fewer as compared to an depth between the LT1 and LT2 for the identical time period.

This way that while the percentage contribution of aerobic lipolysis can be higher at lower intensities, the general quantity of energy derived from aerobic lipolysis may be greater at higher intensities within the same time body.

However, it's miles vital to word that there are obstacles to this. At intensities above the anaerobic threshold and near VO2 max, the bulk of electricity is derived from carbohydrates, with a negligible amount coming from fat.

In conclusion, it's far important to recall that the aerobic electricity device typically operates for the duration of intensities above resting ranges and as a lot as the LT2 factor. The key version arises in the proportions of aerobic lipolysis and aerobic glycolysis, which rely on the exercising intensity. While the ones possibilities alternate, the aerobic electricity tool stays responsible for electricity production inside this range.

Let's flow into on and find out what certainly takes place above the LT2 point. You may additionally additionally have heard that above the LT2 or anaerobic threshold, the aerobic energy device ceases to characteristic, and also you depend totally on the anaerobic glycolytic device for power manufacturing. However, that isn't the case. In reality, the cardio and anaerobic glycolytic energy structures collaborate to generate ATP.

At rest, your frame consumes a specific amount of oxygen to keep its competencies. As you begin to workout, oxygen intake will growth, and the better the depth of on foot, the more the amount of oxygen you're taking in and utilize. Up till the anaerobic threshold, the quantity of oxygen ate up is enough on your frame to provide power aerobically. What happens above the anaerobic threshold is that oxygen intake could no longer lower, however as an alternative continues to growth till attaining the aspect of VO2 max, which represents the maximum amount of oxygen your body can take in.

However, notwithstanding the fact that the oxygen consumption is better than the anaerobic threshold, it is insufficient for muscle companies to completely generate electricity through cardio metabolism. Above the anaerobic threshold depth, the cardio energy machine operates at higher fees because of progressed oxygen usage, especially thru aerobic glycolysis, with a discounted contribution from aerobic lipolysis. The ultimate strength required comes from the anaerobic lactic energy machine, which results in lactate and hydrogen ion accumulation. Simply located, the aerobic machine cannot clear all of the lactate produced due to insufficient oxygen availability, however the extended oxygen intake in assessment to lower intensities.

So, most of the anaerobic threshold and the VO2 max intensities there is a mixture of each aerobic energy, specifically cardio glycolysis, and anaerobic glycolytic electricity.

The last important marker is the VO2 max, and now we're going to discover what takes region with the energy systems past this point. As noted earlier than, at the price much like the VO2 max, your body gets the most quantity of oxygen it is capable of. Beyond 100% of the VO2 max, there can be an oxygen plateau. Therefore, in case you keep walking at a quicker speed than the VO2 max velocity, you may however devour the identical quantity of oxygen as you probably did at your VO2 max velocity. This shows that the aerobic strength tool continues to characteristic and works truly as intensely as at the 100% VO2 max depth, depending heavily on cardio glycolysis for power production, with a minimum contribution, if any, from cardio lipolysis. However, due to the fact the jogging pace is now quicker than the fee associated with the VO2 max, the power desires are higher. Despite the identical oxygen consumption as earlier than, the extended power requirements result in a more reliance at the anaerobic lactic tool compared to the VO2 max depth, as a manner to satisfy the frame's strength needs. In truth, intensities above the VO2 max are especially appropriate for maximum reliable improvement of the anaerobic lactic power machine. While the anaerobic glycolytic system operates above the anaerobic threshold factor, the higher the speed increases beyond the anaerobic threshold, the more tremendous the manufacturing of anaerobic lactic strength becomes, particularly beyond the VO2 max issue, wherein oxygen consumption does now not boom past the only hundred% VO2 max intensity.

In truth, the ones intensities are those that motive the most muscle burning sensation and fatigue, in particular inside the 800m and 400m runs, and to a lesser amount, the 1500m run, all of which can be above the VO2 max depth. Considering the racing times of high-degree athletes, the 3km race is related to the speed much like the VO2 max. Therefore, the 1500m and shorter distance races have speeds that exceed the depth of one hundred% VO2 max, as formerly stated. For people with a slower tempo, the 8-minute walking pace is the velocity associated with the VO2 max. Consequently, any race finished in masses less than 7-eight minutes is above the VO2 max depth.

The higher production of anaerobic glycolytic power related to those races results in a fast buildup of metabolic byproducts, together with hydrogen ions, which increase acidity for your muscle cells and blood, and are liable for muscular fatigue, specially in the 400m and 800m activities. On the possibility hand, in occasions which might be above the anaerobic threshold, but underneath the VO2 max, the anaerobic glycolytic machine even though competencies, but at lower fees in comparison to intensities beyond the VO2 max. As a end result, the accumulation of hydrogen ions takes area extra slowly and to a lesser volume than inside the 400m, 800m, and even the 1500m races.

I would really like to phrase right right here that while oxygen intake remains the identical at intensities above the VO2 max as compared to the VO2 max intensity, and the speeds are higher, there is every other component that influences the extended contribution from anaerobic lactic power. Previously, I defined the complete approach assuming that someone runs at his VO2 max pace after if you want to growth his pace to higher ranges. In this case, the most quantity of oxygen he can intake is to be had for utilization. However, in workout, matters do now not artwork exactly on this manner.

In all races, you begin from a standstill, which means that that on the begin of any of the aforementioned races, you do no longer reap the maximum oxygen consumption you're capable of proper away. The body calls for a while to increase its oxygen uptake while transitioning from a desk sure function to a brief on foot pace. As we referred to earlier, it takes about 1.5-2 mins to benefit maximum oxygen uptake at the velocity associated with 100% VO2 max intensity.

However, at speeds quicker than the most effective associated with the VO2 max (an all-out eight-minute attempt), the VO2 max is reached in much less than 1.Five-2 minutes. For instance, in a 4-minute all-out attempt, maximum oxygen intake can be reached after 1 minute, and in accordance to research on the 800m race, VO2 max is achieved at spherical forty five seconds. In the case of the 400m race, VO2 max is probably reached even faster because of the higher taking walks pace. While I do no longer have the perfect time, I presume it might be round 30 seconds or slightly lower.

So, while you will in the end collect most oxygen consumption in a few unspecified time inside the destiny inside the direction of these races, and that component may be reached earlier than for the duration of slower strolling speeds, it is essential to study that within the preliminary seconds or minutes at the identical time as your oxygen supply stays low, the anaerobic lactic metabolism will perform at its maximum viable charge. However, it does no longer paintings in isolation, and cardio metabolism is constantly involved, albeit to a lesser volume because of decrease oxygen intake. As you method your VO2 max, aerobic metabolism plays a greater massive function.

Thus, the belief is that even above the VO2 max, there may be a aggregate of aerobic and anaerobic lactic strength structures, with a greater contribution from the anaerobic lactic electricity tool in assessment to intensities at or underneath the VO2 max. In terms of the aerobic device's contribution, it plays a comparable position as it does at the intensity of the VO2 max, starting from the aspect wherein you purchased your maximum oxygen uptake. Prior so far, you rely an awful lot less at the cardio device and further at the anaerobic glycolytic device.

Now, after analyzing how strength is produced at severa on foot intensities, let's examine the table below, which illustrates the contribution of strength structures in some unspecified time inside the future of first rate races.

Older tables often suggest higher opportunities of anaerobic contribution for all races above. However, the odds displayed in this desk had been determined based completely mostly on measurements recorded throughout simulated races. It is be conscious that the better the intensity of the race, the more the contribution of the anaerobic tool. However, as you could observe, the strength systems artwork on the aspect of each specific in most instances.

The key take away from this desk is the massive amount of strength provided via manner of the cardio device in most races, which consist of the 800m race. For expert athletes who complete the 800m race in a good deal a whole lot much less than 2 minutes, there has been a misconception that the 800m is regularly an anaerobic glycolytic event. However, this belief is a long way from the reality. Without a well-advanced cardio device, traditional performance within the 800m race might be extensively impaired.

At this issue, I want to emphasize that the contribution of energy systems need to not be determined definitely by using race distance, but as an alternative with the useful resource of race length. This is an important consideration to maintain in mind. For instance, if people run at most strive for five minutes, regardless of the truth that their blanketed distances range considerably, the contribution of the strength systems might be similar for each runners. Despite the discrepancy in distance covered, the strength gadget contributions might be comparable among them because the period of try is the same.

Conversely, while evaluating a expert athlete and a interest jogger inside the 1500m distance, the electricity structures' contribution couldn't be the same. The athlete also can entire the race in beneath three minutes and forty or 45 seconds, whereas the interest jogger might probable require more time. Consequently, the strength production among those efforts may range. The athlete might likely rely greater on his/her anaerobic power tool compared to the interest jogger, who might probable want greater time to complete the 1500m distance. Therefore, the relationship among time and distance is essential even as organizing education, and I will communicate this in greater element later, explaining why it is definitely useful to base your training on time in location of kilometers. For this motive, I actually have blanketed the desk beneath, which illustrates how strength is shipped among aerobic and anaerobic metabolism in step with time, in choice to distance.

Please be conscious that for every race length, the attempt must be most indoors that particular time period to make certain the accuracy of the mentioned chances. Additionally, it is critical to study the extensive contribution of the cardio device in a maximum strive race lasting 75 seconds. This highlights the critical feature of a well-advanced cardio device in activities from 800m and above, as I stated earlier.

Even in a 400m race, a few diploma of aerobic tool improvement is wanted, despite the fact that now not to the identical extent as within the 800m. However, this is predicated upon at the volume of each athlete. For example, a international-magnificence male 400m runner with a time spherical forty 3-40 four seconds in most instances is based totally totally on their anaerobic energy structures with a few guide from their cardio system. On the alternative hand, a girl international-class athlete may additionally moreover require 48-40 nine seconds to complete the race, ensuing in a extra production of cardio power. For slower 400m runs lasting between 50-60 seconds, the proportion contributions shift again, with an multiplied reliance on cardio metabolism.

Therefore, the belief is that in maximum strolling intensities and racing intervals, there can be constantly a combination of energy systems. Some exceptions are prolonged distances like the marathon and half marathon, in which the cardio energy gadget is accountable for close to a hundred% of energy production, even in elite athletes whose instances are shorter than recreational runners. The cutting-edge-day-day 1/2 of marathon international report stands at 57 mins and 31 seconds, a length that corresponds to the anaerobic threshold, that is the maximum point wherein electricity manufacturing is purely generated thru cardio metabolism.

Another exception is sports that very last a lot much less than 10 seconds, which incorporates the jumping and throwing occasions in track and area, further to the 100m race for expert athletes who whole it in 10 seconds or plenty less. In those times, the important energy device is the anaerobic alactic system, which depletes its reserves after a maximum strive of 10 seconds. Lactate manufacturing starts offevolved to boom after spherical 5-6 seconds, but now not extensively as compared to sports much like the 400m and 800m races. And for durations between the extremes of the marathon/half of marathon and the 100m sprint, a aggregate of all the strength systems comes into play, and the contribution of each tool depends on the depth and length of the try.

In remaining, I would like to make a connection with organisation sports sports sports activities regarding the energy structures. While institution sports activities sports are not the primary interest of this ebook, it's miles essential to recognize that the principle energy systems used in some unspecified time in the future of a in shape, whether or not or no longer it's football, basketball, or team handball, are the cardio and anaerobic alactic power structures, now not the anaerobic lactic tool as many assume. These sports activities activities require significant quantities of strength from the alactic metabolism for quick bursts of electricity which includes jumps and short sprints, in addition to a properly-advanced cardio gadget to fast refill the phosphocreatine utilized by the alactic device. If the cardio tool is not nicely advanced, a player will rely upon the anaerobic glycolytic electricity for the short moves of the game because of the reality the cardio gadget will not top off the alactic building blocks brief enough. This reliance at the lactic anaerobic strength gadget will result in fatigue and slower moves compared to the extra effective alactic machine.

Furthermore, a poorly advanced cardio gadget manner that the price at the anaerobic threshold can be low, which interprets to the athlete stepping into the combined aerobic-anaerobic place above the anaerobic threshold in advance than an athlete with a properly-advanced aerobic gadget. This untimely shift to better intensity power structures will result in fatigue. Conversely, a properly-advanced aerobic and alactic tool will permit group exercise gamers to perform fast and powerful actions at some degree within the whole activity with out experiencing immoderate fatigue.

Coaches who teach institution undertaking game enthusiasts with the thoughts-set of treating them like 400m and 800m runners must re-evaluate their training approach straight away. It is critical to apprehend that institution recreation players, regardless of the unique sport, do no longer engage in non-prevent running at most effort for distances like 200m, 300m, or 400m all through a endeavor. Instead, their moves contain a mixture of quick bursts of leaping or sprinting, observed through intervals of taking walks at submaximal aerobic intensities.

Chapter 4: Body's Adaptations To Training

Training consequences in versions related to each strength tool, which can be categorized the ones as cardio, anaerobic lactic and anaerobic alactic permutations.

AEROBIC ADAPTATIONS

Aerobic diversifications can be categorised into precious and peripheral variations. Central variations get up inside the coronary coronary heart and blood, even as peripheral variations take location in the muscle fibers.

CENTRAL ADAPTATIONS

The essential crucial variations embody the subsequent:

1. Increase in stroke amount at relaxation and in some unspecified time

in the future of exercising: Stroke quantity refers to the quantity of blood ejected from the left ventricle of the coronary coronary heart with every heartbeat, measured in milliliters in step with beat. Through training, stroke quantity will boom each at relaxation and for the duration of exercise in contrast to pre-education ranges. This increase method that the coronary heart pumps extra blood with each beat, delivering greater oxygen to the frame. The rise in stroke amount is attributed to modifications in coronary coronary coronary heart period that arise with education. The key diversifications inside the coronary coronary coronary heart that make a contribution to its hypertrophy are the subsequent:

A. Internal dimensions of the left ventricle increase, permitting more blood to fill the ventricle in advance than it is pumped out for circulate.

B. Muscular walls of the heart, specially inside the left ventricle, become thicker, essential to more powerful contractions.

These variations are responsible for the improved stroke quantity. The enlarged length of the coronary coronary heart permits the left ventricle to stretch similarly, accommodating more blood. The extended thickness of the muscular partitions complements contractility, resulting in a more potent pump, allowing the coronary coronary heart to propel extra blood into pass.

2. Resting coronary coronary heart fee decreases: The boom of stroke extent at rest, consequences in a decrease resting coronary coronary coronary heart fee due to the truth more blood is sent with each heartbeat and as a quit end result

the coronary heart doesn't need to conquer as fast, as earlier than the ones diversifications passed off so that you can cowl the frame's desires for oxygen.

Note: While the resting coronary coronary heart rate decreases with schooling, the maximal coronary coronary coronary heart charge doesn't trade with schooling.

three. Increased Cardiac Output at the identical enormous type of heartbeats in assessment to an untrained country: Cardiac output refers to the amount of blood pumped with the aid of the use of the coronary heart in a unmarried minute and is calculated via way of the use of multiplying stroke quantity and coronary heart charge. It is stated in liters consistent with minute. With training, stroke amount will growth, number one to an extended cardiac output at any given heart fee as compared to pre-education levels. This way that irrespective of taking walks intensity, whether or not it is slow or at maximal coronary coronary coronary heart charge, the cardiac output could be extra after the schooling period.

However, there are differing critiques regarding the relationship amongst cardiac output and coronary coronary coronary heart charge at some stage in workout. Some argue that once accomplishing spherical sixty five%-70% of maximum coronary heart fee, cardiac output will boom best thru a better form of heartbeats in step with minute and not due to an boom in stroke quantity. This claim is primarily based totally on earlier studies, which advised that stroke volume plateaus once the coronary coronary heart charge exceeds this threshold. The purpose become that the coronary heart contractions grow to be too speedy to permit enough time for the chambers of the coronary heart to fill with blood.

While it's far actual that those consequences had been located in the mentioned test, subsequent studies has reexamined this trouble and shed more moderate at the conduct of stroke extent throughout exercise. Most researchers have concluded that the stroke extent plateau takes place regularly in untrained people, or even among them, no longer all revel in it. In evaluation, professional staying energy individuals typically have a tendency to showcase a linear growth in stroke amount with coronary heart price till attaining maximum coronary coronary heart rate. Therefore, it's far doubtful that nicely-educated staying strength trainees get maintain of substantial cardiac blessings at sixty 5%-

70% in their most coronary coronary heart price or at decrease on foot intensities. Additionally, it have to be stated that some findings advise that the plateau phenomenon does no longer stand up in untrained humans both.

Note: While the cardiac output of an character increases even as comparing it at the same coronary heart fees in educated and untrained states, it stays unchanged at relaxation, maintaining the equal levels as in advance than a person started training. This happens because of the truth cardiac output is the end result of beats in line with minute superior with the useful aid of stroke quantity (beats everyday with minute x stroke quantity). As stroke quantity will growth at any given coronary heart fee, the cardiac output may also growth for that specific coronary coronary coronary heart price. However, whilst in the path of workout, expanded oxygen is important for higher usual performance at some stage in all taking walks intensities, at rest, the body's oxygen needs do now not trade. A precise quantity of oxygen is actually required for each day physical capabilities. As referred to in advance, a expert character's coronary coronary heart can meet the frame's oxygen goals with fewer beats regular with minute due to the increased stroke quantity.

In less tough phrases, in case your resting coronary heart rate earlier than training end up sixty four beats in step with minute, the elevated stroke volume because of education now lets in a bigger cardiac output at sixty four beats in keeping with minute. Consequently, the heart can now meet the body's oxygen goals with fewer beats in keeping with minute, permit's say fifty beats as an example. Thus, the cardiac output at fifty beats steady with minute is equal to the preceding output at sixty four beats constant with minute.

4. Increase inside the pink blood cells and hemoglobin levels: Endurance schooling can purpose an boom in pink blood cellular and hemoglobin tiers. Red blood cells incorporate hemoglobin, and having a better rely of each can appreciably benefit staying electricity typical performance. This is due to the truth that hemoglobin lets in the transportation of oxygen throughout the frame, resulting in a complicated oxygen-sporting capability.

PERIPHERAL ADAPTATIONS

1. Increased capillary density round muscle fibers: Capillaries are blood vessels decided at some degree within the frame that play a essential position in transporting blood, vitamins, and oxygen

to cells in severa organ and body structures. They can be considered due to the reality the 'stop of the road' in the frame's vascular community. With the growth of the capillary community surrounding muscle fibers, the transport of oxygen and vitamins to the muscle businesses will even growth. Additionally, capillaries resource inside the removal of waste products from the muscle tissue.

In plenty less complicated phrases, the boom in muscle capillary density due to patience education has key benefits. Firstly, it lets in for extra uptake of oxygen via the muscular tissues, thereby improving ordinary overall performance. Secondly, it allows a quicker restore and healing technique via the usage of manner of improving the elimination of waste merchandise.

2. Increase within the giant range and density of mitochondria: Mitochondria are microscopic, membrane-positive organelles determined in most cells of the body, besides for purple blood cells. Muscle cells, particularly, comprise hundreds or maybe masses of mitochondria because of their immoderate power needs. These organelles are frequently called the 'powerhouse of the cellular' because of the truth their primary function is aerobic energy manufacturing. Within muscle cells, mitochondria play a crucial position in breaking down nutrients ate up inside the presence of oxygen (cardio metabolism) to generate the power desired for exercise, as we referred to in the evaluation of the aerobic strength tool. In smooth phrases, mitochondria make use of the oxygen we breathe and the nutrients we consume to deliver ATP

(adenosine triphosphate), this is the electricity foreign cash of the frame.

So, how does this relate to walking or each other persistence pastime? The presence of more mitochondria lets in for a higher production of ATP thru cardio metabolism all through workout. The extra the quantity of ATP produced with the resource of manner of your cells, the more power you want to run longer and quicker, allowing you to undergo for prolonged intervals.

Note: While mitochondria can produce ATP within the presence of oxygen, and cardio power manufacturing occurs inside them, this doesn't endorse that jogging intensities related to anaerobic performance do now not enhance from a complicated number and density of mitochondria. As we've got were given seen earlier, the aerobic electricity tool performs a big position in various sports activities sports activities and running intensities, and the cardio and anaerobic structures normally artwork together in maximum instances.

three. Increases inside the degrees of aerobic enzymes within the mitochondria: This model goes hand in hand with will boom inside the massive variety and density of mitochondria. An growth in mitochondria leads to an growth in cardio enzymes interior them, and vice versa. This interprets to a better manufacturing of strength-ATP inside the presence of oxygen, as we referred to earlier. Essentially, the increase in cardio enzymes within the mitochondria, combined with the boom inside the variety and density of mitochondria, can be categorized as a single version.

4. More muscle fibers adapt for aerobic endurance overall performance: The muscle consists of three special varieties of muscle fibers: slow twitch fibers or kind 1, and rapid twitch fibers which may be in addition labeled into rapid twitch 2B and rapid twitch 2A fibers.

Slow twitch, type 1 fibers do no longer settlement as forcefully as the short twitch fibers, but they've got a super functionality to provide strength for extended durations due to their reliance on aerobic respiratory to generate ATP. However, their power era functionality is especially decrease than that of rapid twitch fibers.

On the opportunity hand, kind 2B muscle fibers are the maximum effective and most explosive most of the three sorts, but they have confined persistence capacity and broadly talking rely on anaerobic metabolism.

Type 2A fibers very own tendencies of every sluggish twitch and fast twitch 2B fibers. In a muscle biopsy, we might test natural purple muscle fibers representing gradual twitch type 1, and herbal white fibers representing rapid twitch 2B. Between the ones extremes, there are numerous shades of each purple and white, representing the fast twitch 2A fibers. These fibers exhibit a mix of cardio capability, even though no longer as cautioned as sluggish twitch fibers, and the ability to agreement forcefully, regardless of the truth that no longer as explosively as rapid twitch 2B fibers. Consequently, they're capable of the use of every cardio and anaerobic respiratory.

Regarding the conversion of muscle fibers thru training, research has shown that gradual twitch fibers do not transform into speedy twitch fibers. Instead, what takes location with education is a conversion of fast twitch fibers from type 2B to kind 2A, and this alteration occurs regardless of the form of schooling finished. Whether sporting out lengthy aerobic periods or dash and energy education, studies endorse that the conversion from 2B to 2A fibers takes region.

It may additionally moreover moreover seem ordinary that during spite of quick, maximal sprint training, which carefully makes use of 2B fibers, this conversion nevertheless occurs. However, studies continuously allows this phenomenon. The equal applies to energy schooling and really each specific type of training. Interestingly, at the same time as a person is sedentary, he/she has a tendency to have more 2B fibers in assessment to his/her educated u . S ., no matter the specific training habitual he/she undertakes. This version might serve to enhance muscle restoration and allow better patience during schooling strain due to the fact Type 2A fibers showcase greater fatigue resistance in comparison to 2B fibers. Athletes with a higher percentage of intermediate fibers relative to 2B fibers have a propensity to experience advanced restoration amongst periods and excessive efforts interior a exercising.

Another phenomenon which could occur in muscle fibers, mainly in kind 2A fibers, is their functionality to accumulate developments of either sluggish twitch or speedy twitch fibers counting on the sort of schooling an individual undertakes. For instance, in endurance athletes, type

2A fibers may moreover display off more slow twitch developments, making them better proper for aerobic respiratory. On the opportunity hand, in quick dash athletes which include 100m or 200m sprinters, kind 2A fibers can also show extra forcefulness and a choice for anaerobic respiration.

These variations in muscle fiber types have top notch implications for aerobic training. Intermediate rapid twitch 2A fibers can increase staying power dispositions and elevated fatigue resistance. This transformation takes vicinity thru the diversifications previously said. Slow twitch fibers encompass the very excellent attention of mitochondria, even as fast twitch 2A fibers also very own a massive quantity. In evaluation, the herbal white fast twitch 2B fibers include minimal, if any, mitochondria, ensuing in decrease fatigue resistance.

Therefore, growing the kind of mitochondria and enhancing aerobic enzymes within as many muscle fibers as viable consequences in a more green cardio energy device.

Chapter 5: Anaerobic-Lactic Adaptations

Compared to aerobic variations, anaerobic lactic diversifications have a significantly restrained ability for development. Typically, those permutations can be maximized within a period of 4 to 6 weeks. While cardio basic usual performance is predicated upon on oxygen delivery and uptake, anaerobic familiar common performance is inspired via extra honest factors.

The genetic difficulty furthermore plays a huge feature. The proportion of rapid twitch fibers in an character's muscular tissues is closely associated with anaerobic normal performance. For example, an athlete with approximately eighty% slow twitch fibers will no longer outperform an athlete with the opposite share of muscle fibers in anaerobic activities, irrespective of the amount of anaerobic education. It's essential to be conscious that the 80% rate represents an excessive case, and most human beings own muscle fiber sorts in more balanced possibilities.

Now, allow's delve into the anaerobic glycolytic diversifications that occur with education. These diversifications consist of:

1. Increase in hobby and quantity of key glycolytic enzymes: A higher level of enzymes involved in anaerobic glycolysis allows for a extra charge of glucose breakdown into ATP. This multiplied enzymatic interest lets in muscle fibers to generate ATP at a quicker fee, ensuing in extra energy production.

2. Increase within the muscle mass' buffering capability: As we already apprehend, above a powerful strolling

depth, that is the anaerobic threshold, hydrogen ions gather. Depending on the intensity and length of the effort, this accumulation can arise unexpectedly, such as inside the 400m or 800m races, or it is able to take a chunk longer in races much like the 3km and 5km, in which it could not be as brilliant as within the shorter activities.

The accumulation of hydrogen ions motives acidity to your muscle cells and blood, resulting in muscular fatigue, a burning sensation, and interference with muscular contraction. Your frame employs severa buffering mechanisms to sluggish down the buildup of acidity inside the muscle businesses. We can define muscle buffering capacity because the potential of muscle mass to neutralize the acid/hydrogen ions that acquire at some stage in excessive-intensity exercising, thereby delaying the onset of fatigue. However, those mechanisms quality very last for about forty seconds in the course of an all-out attempt. After this component, the acidity within the muscle cells negatively affects muscular contraction, predominant to excessive fatigue. The 40-2nd mark is particular to maximum try. For an lousy lot much less immoderate efforts, fatigue will set in a piece later, relying on the level of exertion. The extra excessive the try, the sooner acidity will rise up within the muscle mass.

As said in advance, variations from anaerobic glycolytic training have restrained functionality for development. While you can quite boom the capability to delay fatigue, if your muscle's buffering capability will boom, you want to no longer anticipate huge performance gains from this form of schooling.

Moreover, it's miles crucial to make smooth a commonplace false impression. Many people partner this model with the capability to face up to extreme feelings of fatigue and muscle pain, or characteristic it to lactate tolerance schooling. However, this association is virtually incorrect. This model within the primary enables your frame produce electricity anaerobically for a barely longer length, correctly delaying the onset of excessive fatigue for a few seconds. Nevertheless, at the equal time as intense fatigue gadgets in, the precept element that permits you to preserve exercise is not the anaerobic tool, the buffering mechanisms, or lactate tolerance, as usually believed. It is, in fact, a properly-developed cardio device.

Whenever the sensation of excessive fatigue emerges, your anaerobic glycolytic gadget reaches its most functionality to generate strength. Athletes with a enormously advanced cardio device have the capability to preserve higher energy outputs beyond this detail as compared to people with underdeveloped aerobic structures. Why is that? Because a well-developed aerobic device strategies the waste products related to muscle acidity at a quicker price than an underdeveloped one. Consequently, you can maintain your pace for an extended length with much less fatigue and less impaired muscular contractions.

It is critical to understand that whilst enhancing anaerobic and buffering capacities can delay the onset of intense fatigue, the muse for sustained simple normal performance lies in developing a strong aerobic machine.

CONCLUSION

The backside line is that even as a few variations arise for the anaerobic glycolytic tool's fashionable performance, the ones permutations are restricted and can be maximized fairly fast.

Interestingly, electricity education may offer more overall performance profits for this device compared to the two variations said in advance. By developing maximal power, athletes can generate extra stress into the ground, enhancing their regular strength output. When mixed with unique anaerobic schooling tailored to the person's workout, widespread standard overall performance upgrades can be completed. It is actually worth noting that the variations of electricity and aerobic capability are the satisfactory ones that take years to extend and feature lengthy-lasting consequences. Aerobic staying strength and maximal energy function the inspiration for masses awesome sports activities sports. Some sports activities activities require more emphasis on power, while others prioritize persistence.

The drawback, but, is that electricity training can purpose an boom in muscular weight for runners, which can be unfavourable to performance due to the truth large muscle groups require greater oxygen. Therefore, at the same time as I do not forget energy schooling to be important for education in the 400m event and shorter distances, I accept as true with that for distances of 800m and above, interest should be directed in the direction of different factors of schooling. It is proper that energy education can assist an 800m runner growth anaerobic energy, but as I in fact have emphasised earlier than, accomplishing proper times in the 800m with out a well-superior cardio device is really now not possible. In such instances, people have to carefully weigh the specialists and cons in advance than figuring out whether or now not to include electricity education in an 800m software.

I receive as true with that the electricity thing for an 800m athlete can be successfully blanketed via hill sprints, which permits for a better stability with other training components. Hill sprints may not provide the identical maximal strength earnings as weight training, however they may be less bodily annoying and do no longer bring about weight advantage like conventional power schooling.

The claim that you can bring together strength with out inclusive of weight is without a doubt a fantasy that has continued for many years. Apart from the initial period of neural income in the first few weeks of weight education, in which the body learns the actions and muscle synchronization, power gains regularly stand up through muscle increase, which can be unfavourable to runners in distances of 800m and above. The 400m event is a certainly one of a type story, wherein most pace, energy, and electricity are the proscribing factors.

A very last be aware on energy training for staying power-educated people: If you make a decision to include energy training into your regimen, it is essential to keep away from doing immoderate repetitions (15 or 20 reps) to assemble muscular persistence, as many staying power fans generally usually have a tendency to do. The particular persistence preferred for your runs can be superior through your schooling plan and walking itself. Weight education instructions should attention on increasing power, in preference to staying power. The shorter the space of a race, the more incredible the location of maximal power turns into.

I won't delve further into the issue of electricity education as it's far beyond the scope of this ebook. For the ones inquisitive about studying extra about power education, I advocate locating out my specific e-book titled "Natural Muscles: Maximize Your Strength and Muscle Mass Naturally with Just 2 Weight Training Sessions in keeping with

Week." While it extra frequently than no longer caters to humans searching out to bring together a muscular body genuinely, it covers diverse topics together with the mind of electricity improvement, the function of muscle fibers during special repetition stages, techniques for progressing strength, and dispelling common myths surrounding this kind of training.

ANAEROBIC-ALACTIC ADAPTATIONS

What applies to the anaerobic lactic device concerning its room for version also applies proper here, however to a fair greater extent. The alactic device has the least room from development among all three strength systems.

An person with a immoderate percentage of rapid-twitch fibers generally has a more nicely-advanced alactic strength system. This is because of the truth fast-twitch fibers can store a considerably huge amount of phosphocreatine compared to slow-twitch fibers. Phosphocreatine is a crucial element for ATP production inside the alactic gadget, and the more the quantity of phosphocreatine within the muscle businesses, the more electricity can be made from this device and for a slightly longer length. However, as soon as the phosphocreatine stores are depleted, this tool can not generate any greater strength. While creatine dietary dietary supplements are commonly used, they may be able to best increase phosphocreatine stores to a restricted volume and no longer considerably. Both alactic schooling and creatine supplementation can't dramatically increase phosphocreatine stores.

An athlete can gain more universal overall performance gains in phrases of strength outputs within the anaerobic systems thru will growth in maximal strength in contrast to the diversifications as a result of unique schooling for those systems. For sprinters competing in races below 400m, the combination of maximal energy training and maximal sprinting is the recommended training approach. Maximal energy schooling lets in the era of excessive strain outputs with every step on the ground, at the same time as maximal pace schooling complements the charge of pressure development with each step. By combining the ones education components, common ordinary overall performance can decorate, especially within the direction of acceleration levels wherein floor contact instances are longer, bearing in mind the application of extra strength. It is essential to be conscious that maximal tempo, being in big element encouraged by genetics, has a wonderful deal much less capacity for improvement via strength training as compared to the acceleration phase. This is due to the pretty brief ground contact times in the course of maximal speed, which limit the expression of electricity to a lesser quantity. However, income in acceleration can reason progressed not unusual race instances from 100m to 400m activities. It's well well worth mentioning that the ones improvements can also bring about a most discount of 1-2 seconds for really untrained people in a 100m race, and tenths of a 2d for exceedingly knowledgeable athletes. Therefore, the phrase 'sprinters are born and marathoners are made' holds right, in particular considering the frame's variations to training.

Chapter 6: Determinants Of Endurance Performance

Endurance can be generally characterised because of the reality the capacity to maintain a particular tempo or energy output over an extended time frame. The overall overall performance of staying strength sports is based widely speakme on factors: VO2 max and on foot financial system.

VO2 MAX

As we already apprehend, VO2 max represents the maximum extent of oxygen the frame can devour in line with minute. VO2 max may be expressed each in absolute or relative terms. Relative VO2 max is measured as milliliters of oxygen constant with kilogram of body weight constant with minute (ml/kg/min). On the alternative hand, absolute VO2 max does not keep in mind an character's weight and is expressed as milliliters of oxygen consistent with minute (ml/min). In weight-bearing sports activities sports like strolling, institution sports activities activities, and martial arts, wherein the body goals to triumph over gravity, the relative VO2 max is of extra importance. Conversely, in non-weight-bearing sports activities consisting of biking, rowing, and swimming, in which the frame is supported via wheels or water and there can be no gravity to overcome, genuinely the charge of VO2 max is more large. Therefore, at the same time as referring to VO2 max as regards to on foot, we cognizance completely at the relative rate.

There is a big debate surrounding the main limiting elements of VO2 max. One mind-set argues that imperative or oxygen transport diversifications are the important factors, while others suggest that peripheral or oxygen utilization permutations play a larger position in identifying VO2 max levels and development.

After huge research on the hassle, it's far indicated that the number one factors influencing VO2 max stages are the essential permutations. This technique that the diversifications associated with the transport of oxygen to the frame's tissues, which encompass the coronary heart's capability to pump blood and a excessive oxygen-sporting potential due to sufficient red blood cellular be counted and hemoglobin tiers, decide the amount to which VO2 max may be superior. The maximum large proscribing component is the coronary coronary heart's pumping quantity, known as stroke extent, and the associated cardiac hypertrophy changes, making it the maximum vital edition for growing VO2 max.

VO2 max is accomplished at the most coronary coronary coronary heart charge. While most coronary coronary heart rate does not exchange with schooling, an growth in stroke amount, which represents the quantity of blood the heart pumps with every beat, effects in a better cardiac output (stroke quantity × coronary coronary heart beats in step with minute). This, in flip, consequences in a more amount of blood being pumped at maximal coronary heart fees, most vital to a higher VO2 max.

In addition to extended stroke quantity, weight loss can also make a contribution to improvements in relative VO2 max, because the relative price is calculated with an man or woman's weight factored in. Conversely, weight benefit decreases relative VO2 max, which ought to be avoided for best patience ordinary overall performance.

In phrases of improvement capability, VO2 max can be improved thru training as it's far encouraged by means of the usage of manner of key training variations. However, in contrast to the development of strolling financial machine, VO2 max has plenty much less room for improvement, and genetic factors play a massive function. On common, people can count on an boom in VO2 max of spherical 20% with training. However, there have been recorded instances of enhancements as a great deal as 30%, and in rare intense times, whilst a good deal as forty%-50%, even though such instances are uncommon.

RUNNING ECONOMY

While VO2 max is an vital factor of staying energy standard performance, and no longer a vain one, as endorsed thru a few coaches, strolling economic system is similarly crucial and, in fact, even greater vital for achieving proper staying electricity ordinary overall performance.

Running economic machine refers to the amount of oxygen your frame requires to preserve a specific pace at the equal time as on foot. The lower your oxygen consumption at that tempo, the higher your on foot monetary machine becomes. For instance, permit's undergo in thoughts an individual who runs at a tempo of 12 km/h, which corresponds to eighty% of hisVO2 max. At this depth, he consumes eighty% of his most oxygen consumption constant with minute. However, through regular training, the character improves his going for walks monetary machine and maintain the same 12 km/h pace at simplest 75% of his VO2 max. This manner he can maintain the same speed on the equal time as requiring an awful lot less oxygen, assuming his VO2 max stays unchanged. It's essential to phrase that if his VO2 max did increase, his oxygen consumption at 75% of his VO2 max may be higher than his previous seventy five% VO2 max. However, a reduction in oxygen requirements at a given tempo indicates an development in walking economic device. Alternatively, this development method that the individual can preserve a faster tempo at the same time as maintaining the same stage of oxygen intake he previously had whilst on foot at 12 km/h.

So, how can someone preserve a quicker tempo with the equal oxygen intake as earlier than or run on the equal velocity however with heaps much less want for oxygen?

This development pertains to muscular peripheral variations. The extra mitochondria and aerobic enzymes your muscle groups have, the greater successfully they could utilize the oxygen added via your circulatory tool. Before those muscular variations rise up, your circulatory tool elements the same amount of oxygen, however your muscular gadget is not as able to efficiently accepting and utilising large quantities of it. After the permutations take location, you could now utilize more quantities of oxygen despatched from your circulatory device. This technique that you can run quicker at the equal VO2 max percent, or you can run on the equal velocity as in advance than however at a decrease percent of your maximum oxygen consumption.

Ultimately, this example demonstrates the essence of staying power training enhancements.

When a person is untrained and begins offevolved on foot, he is going to reach higher probabilities of his VO2 max at sluggish speeds. As he adapts to education over time, he can be able to keep the identical velocity at decrease possibilities of VO2 max, resulting in lower coronary coronary heart expenses. For instance, initially, he may also run at seventy five% of his VO2 max or at a coronary coronary heart charge of 80 five% - 86% of his most, which corresponds to seventy five% of VO2 max, at a pace of 10 km/h. After some time, his coronary heart fee will drop to 80% of his most, further to the share of VO2 max, on the identical going for walks pace. As a result, he's able to cowl greater distance at the identical possibilities of VO2 max and most heart fee in evaluation to on the equal time as he started out out schooling.

Besides the peripheral permutations, which may be the number one elements contributing to better jogging economic gadget via inexperienced oxygen utilization, it appears that evidently the interplay of numerous biomechanical variables moreover plays a function. However, no unmarried issue of these variables has a giant effect on taking walks financial system.

Certain anthropometric trends, which encompass extended, slender legs with a majority of mass dispensed better on the thigh, a slim pelvis, and small toes, appear to make contributions to advanced taking walks financial gadget. These elements, associated with an character's frame construct and mass distribution, can provide advantages; however, they can't be changed through education.

Additionally, jogging form plays a function in running monetary system. Runners who display off much less vertical oscillation (decreased bouncing while strolling) will be inclined to have higher walking monetary device. Over time, with training, runners instinctively and unconsciously expand the most maximum suitable strolling shape to maximize overall performance. Furthermore, various styles of education, which include rapid on foot consisting of strides, sprints, c program languageperiod education, hill schooling, plyometrics, and strength schooling, will have a high-quality impact on taking walks form. These education techniques help muscle groups lessen wasted motion, cast off vain movements, and keep manage at high speeds. The enhancements received from speedy-velocity training translate to better strolling shape and reduced wasted movement at slower speeds. As a give up result, lots lots less strength and oxygen are required to propel the body forward, most important to improved taking walks financial device at some stage in precise speeds and intensities.

However, it is essential no longer to be burdened. No depend how fast you run to your education, sizable earnings in walking economic gadget can not be expected with out the improvement of muscular peripheral variations thru aerobic training. All the quick walking physical activities are absolutely complementary factors that can decorate your going for walks monetary system to a point. The actual upgrades in on foot monetary tool come from constant cardio sessions. It's as smooth as that and might not need to be more complicated. I accept as actual with many people normally normally generally tend to overanalyze the concept of on foot monetary gadget and pass over the bigger photograph. They attempt to incorporate severa variables into the improvement of walking financial system, on the identical time as, in reality, it's far pretty easy. The key factors that enhance taking walks financial system are right within the front of our eyes, however many forget them. It regularly involves splendid amounts of aerobic education to maximise the improvement of muscular peripheral versions, along incorporating some speedy on foot sports, which play a smaller function in improving on foot shape and coordination at slower speeds. That's all it takes.

Chapter 7: Fractional Utilization

Fractional usage of VO2 max is a third variable that affects staying power basic overall performance. It represents the proportion of VO2 max that may be sustained in a few unspecified time within the future of a race. VO2 max is the maximum quantity of oxygen that your body can eat. Different walking intensities beneath the rate related to VO2 max correspond to particular possibilities of VO2 max. The ability to preserve a better percent of VO2 max at submaximal intensities is beneficial for commonplace performance as it permits for added oxygen utilization and, consequently, accelerated aerobic power manufacturing.

For example, the anaerobic threshold of amateur staying power-skilled people is commonly around seventy five% of VO2 max, which corresponds to about eighty five% of their most coronary coronary heart price. Through training, an athlete can enhance and push the brink difficulty to stand up at spherical 80%-eighty five% of VO2 max, correlated with a heart price type of 88%-ninety two% of his most coronary coronary heart price. This improvement technique that during his one-hour maximum on foot pace, this is the pace on the anaerobic threshold, he may be capable of consume extra oxygen below clearly cardio conditions, ensuing in quicker race instances.

However, this improvement can display up quite quicker than the improvement of strolling economic system. After a powerful education length, the bulk of endurance-educated humans fall in the type of 88% to ninety two% in their most coronary coronary heart charge in regard to the anaerobic threshold coronary heart fee. No one may have an anaerobic threshold lots higher than ninety % in their most coronary heart charge. Please examine that I stated "a extraordinary deal higher." While a few athletes may additionally moreover have an anaerobic threshold slightly above the ninety % mark, those instances are exceptions. Anything past this factor is an exception and not the rule. If it does arise, it is going to be handiest barely above the ninety two% coronary heart fee mark. Anaerobic thresholds at coronary coronary coronary heart charges of ninety 5%, 96%, or 90 seven% of the maximum in reality do no longer exist.

So, the bottom line is that novice human beings are able to maintain a lower percentage of their VO2 max in comparison to properly-educated athletes for the identical period of time. However, as they adapt and improvement with their schooling, it appears that all nicely-professional individuals will be predisposed to run at comparable chances in their VO2 max if their race instances are comparable.

For instance, if one individual desires 50 mins to finish a 10km race, he goes to not be strolling on the identical percent of VO2 max as an individual who completes the 10km race in half of-hour. The slower person can be taking walks at a decrease percentage of VO2 max. However, among those who quit the race inside the equal or similar time, their fractional usage of VO2 max might be greater or plenty much less comparable.

How does this improvement take place?

With the identical variations that walking financial gadget is advanced. More mitochondria, more aerobic enzymes, and better capillary density bring about better cardio energy manufacturing at better possibilities of VO2max because of the truth well-superior muscular adaptations are accountable for getting rid of metabolic waste products. The greater of those versions there are (mitochondria, cardio enzymes, capillaries), the more efficiently aerobic metabolism can upward push up at higher intensities.

Keep in mind, even though, that this improvement cannot keep indefinitely, as everyone can also then be able to run a marathon or half of marathon at one hundred% VO2max. However, after a plateau takes region, going for walks monetary device can although maintain to increase and provide typical overall performance earnings.

THE INTERACTION BETWEEN THE BIG 2 ON ENDURANCE PERFORMANCE

While patience overall performance is predicated on three factors—VO2 max, strolling economic device, and fractional utilization—the 2 number one factors that notably impact persistence performance are walking economic device and VO2 max. While fractional usage does beautify with training, there may be a limit to its non-save you development, as formerly noted. Additionally, among athletes of similar ranges and comparable race instances, fractional usage has a bent to seem at comparable possibilities of VO2 max, without large discrepancies. Consequently, the very last outcomes of a race among athletes with comparable improvement hinges upon their VO2 max and running financial tool, further to the dynamic interplay among those factors.

Let's begin our analysis through that specialize in an person athlete in isolation, without making comparisons to others. This approach will permit us to apprehend the significance of each VO2 max and strolling financial tool and the manner they both play vital roles.

For instance, permit's undergo in thoughts an athlete with a VO2 max of 60 ml/kg/min. On common, the athlete uses the subsequent probabilities of his VO2 max for the duration of specific races:

As you could have located, inside the table above, I in reality have supplied race periods in choice to race distances. This is due to the fact, as said before, the percentage of VO2 max that someone can employ depends extra on time in desire to distance. Additionally, the possibilities referred to above are averages, and with education, maximum humans might be close to those values. That's why I decide upon now not to overanalyze the idea of fractional utilization and get lost inside the records. While it virtually performs a function, and an character who can preserve a greater percent of his VO2 max for an prolonged length will constantly have an advantage, the variations in opportunities are not huge between athletes of similar tiers and times. Therefore, to keep matters easy, with out problems understandable, and not lose sight of the bigger photograph, it's miles higher for us to interest on VO2 max and going for walks financial tool instead of fractional utilization.

If the person noted above will growth his VO2 max from 60 ml/kg/min to 65 ml/kg/min, the amount of oxygen he will eat for the same percent of his VO2 max could be extra. Consequently, he can be capable of produce more power aerobically. Take a glance underneath and have a look at how, with the extended VO2 max, he can now deliver a greater amount of oxygen to his muscle mass at 90 5%, 90%, and eighty five% of his VO2 max as compared to his preceding portions at 100%, 95%, and 90% of his VO2 max, respectively.

Therefore, top values of VO2 max are particularly important, and the higher the rate, the higher. However, an individual can despite the fact that enhance his performance without growing his VO2 max if he consciousness on enhancing his on foot financial machine. Let's keep in thoughts the state of affairs in which the character's VO2 max is at the preliminary price of 60 ml/kg/min. By improving his muscular cardio diversifications, which includes developing the massive sort of mitochondria, aerobic enzymes, and capillary density, he can be in a role to make use of a greater quantity of the brought oxygen for aerobic strength production.

For instance, permit's expect that his circulatory device offers you a sure amount of oxygen for a given intensity. After some schooling, he makes upgrades especially associated with peripheral muscular variations, with none trade in his VO2 max. In this example, his circulatory system will even though delivery the equal amount of oxygen (targeted as X) for the equal intensity. However, his muscular tissues will now have the capacity to make use of a extra percentage of this X amount of oxygen in evaluation to earlier than the muscular variations happened. As a cease end result, while the identical amount of oxygen is being brought, the character is now able to going for walks quicker at the equal intensity because of advanced oxygen utilization. Furthermore, the preceding pace that was sustained at this intensity can now be maintained at a decrease intensity in which the frame gives a lesser quantity of oxygen. This improvement in taking walks monetary tool is accomplished with none alternate within the VO2 max fee.

You understand now why every VO2 max and jogging financial system, or precious variations and peripheral variations, which may be correlated with the 2 factors cited above, are so important. In the above instance, if each VO2 max and walking economic system are advanced concurrently, this athlete will experience greater performance improvements in contrast to each improvement one by one.

So, how do a little coaches claim that VO2 max isn't an vital trouble?

They look at it in isolation and form their opinion based totally on the remark that some athletes with decrease VO2 max values have outperformed humans with better VO2 max values. This remark is honestly real, as there are times in which athletes with decrease VO2 max values gain higher race times as compared to people with better VO2 max. The underlying aspect contributing to this phenomenon is strolling monetary device.

To better recognize this idea, allow's delve right right into a hypothetical instance.

Three runners with same VO2 max values run at ninety% of their VO2 max during a 10km race, resulting inside the same oxygen intake. However, there are variations in their race instances. Athlete 1 completes the race in 36 minutes, Athlete 2 finishes in 38 minutes, and Athlete three requires forty minutes to cover the gap.

So, what determines their instances is their on foot financial system. Athlete 1 has more properly-developed peripheral versions, which help his muscle organizations take delivery of and use oxygen greater successfully. Thus, he's capable of run faster regardless of having the same amount of circulatory oxygen as the opposite athletes. As a stop end result, he also can be capable of run at the speeds that the other athletes run the 10km distance, however at a lower intensity and percentage of VO2 max.

This lower depth and percentage of VO2 max translate to better strolling financial machine. Sure, some super minor factors play a characteristic, which includes form and anthropometry, as I cited during the strolling monetary gadget evaluation. However, the principle trouble proper here is the cardio abilities of the muscle businesses.

Let's have a look at a real-existence example now. Derek Clayton became a runner who set a marathon worldwide record of 2:09:36 in 1967. His VO2 max modified into sixty eight ml/kg/min, and he received the race and set a worldwide report concurrently, in spite of various contributors having higher VO2 maxes. A VO2 max of sixty eight ml/kg/min isn't considered high enough for a marathoner. Many argue that he had a high fractional usage of his VO2 max at some stage in the race. However, fractional usage could not variety substantially among athletes at comparable ranges. What led him to victory and the vicinity file grow to be his walking monetary device and incredibly efficient muscular machine. He correctly carried out any to be had oxygen furnished via way of his coronary coronary coronary heart and blood.

Therefore, as usual usual overall performance differs amongst two human beings with the equal VO2 max due to specific muscular aerobic capabilities, the same precept applies whilst an athlete with a decrease VO2 max defeats an athlete with a better VO2 max. However, this does not advocate that VO2 max tiers hold no rate. In reality, people who've gained races with decrease VO2 maxes than others ought to further beautify their times in the event that they had higher VO2 max tiers.

Both VO2 max and strolling economic device play vital roles in race instances and ordinary staying power of an athlete. In fact, a excessive VO2 max is a prerequisite for being a worldwide-elegance patience athlete. An individual with a VO2 max of fifty ml/kg/min will in no way outperform someone with a VO2 max of 75 ml/kg/min, despite the fact that the previous maximizes his peripheral variations. The difference is definitely too considerable.

However, at the same time as the versions in VO2 max aren't massive, it will become tough to expect the race very last results totally based on VO2 max. Nonetheless, this doesn't lessen the significance of VO2 max. In fact, a higher VO2 max gives a higher ceiling and additional capacity for development. When mixed with maximized peripheral muscular variations, a sufficiently excessive VO2 max becomes a recipe for achieving worldwide-beauty staying power levels.

However, an critical difficulty to maintain in mind is that genetics play a vast position in identifying an individual's VO2 max, and it can't be superior to the identical volume as going for walks monetary device. While each VO2 max and walking economic machine contribute to typical overall performance improvements for novices, extra superior runners may additionally moreover furthermore attain a plateau of their VO2 max. In such cases, similarly performance upgrades are completed via the improvement of jogging economy and the related muscular variations.

Chapter 8: Understanding The Fundamentals

According to research finished with the resource of Yale Medicine, on commonplace spherical 50-sixty five% of runners get injured a yr and while some of the ones injuries can be because of falls or wonderful surprising incidents, the bulk are because of overuse. (Running Injuries, 2022) Overuse happens when the body is not nicely prepared for the strain of the hobby you are asking it to do. For example, the common individual might now not discover themselves signing as plenty as compete in a weightlifting competition without the proper education and guidance in advance of time. It seems clean in those situations in which heavy weights are worried and harm appears plenty extra inevitable without the proper form and muscle groups built up. Similarly, in case you are new to strolling, aiming to growth mileage, or surely getting returned out after a chunk of a hiatus, without the right conditioning you will probably find out yourself injured.

The most crucial gain of flexibleness in runners is joint mobility. Stretching will increase flexibility, which in the long run permits your joints to transport more freely. When the joints can flow into more freely the chance of damage decreases dramatically due to the truth your joints are capable of run thru their entire kind of motion and are not limited via tight muscle corporations and ligaments. It is vital for our joints to transport through their entire kind of movement; in any other case the fluid the body circulates to coat the joint surfaces cannot do its pastime, which results within the joints turning into stiff and visit pot. This deterioration can reason weakened bone shape and arthritis that could purpose a myriad of issues for runners.

This elevated joint mobility no longer nice reduces the threat of damage, weakened bone shape, and arthritis; however it is able to moreover help enhance your universal normal normal performance. When joints can flow into at their complete functionality there is a lot much less resistance that can significantly help boom pace and sturdiness to your strolling.

Most human beings that I really have spoken to which is probably avid runners were given into it because it started out as a handy way to stay in shape, be active, and experience the out of doors. There are not any gym memberships had to run and the overall charges are minimum in evaluation to specific sports. For this purpose, it may seem overwhelming to feature some thing new in your time desk. Thankfully, there are a few very brief smooth steps to increasing flexibility and joint mobility that do not require a good buy introduced effort and time. The key stretches for harm prevention attention at the runner's legs, toes, and lower once more, and there are various approaches to attain these targeted areas.

It is also important to realise at the same time as and the way to stretch correctly based totally on what you're aiming to perform. It also can seem a piece unexpected, however many studies display that stretching proper earlier than a run can reason damage in choice to prevent it. The Mayo Clinic's take a look at indicates that stretching cold muscle organizations can growth the hazard of harm. It also can probable decrease performance if done previous to an excessive exercising, which includes a marathon or music and discipline sports sports. Some research even showed that stretching right away earlier than an event can cause the hamstrings to weaken and emerge as more at risk of fatigue and harm. (Stretching: Focus on Flexibility, 2022)

This does now not endorse that athletes need to hit the ground jogging without any heat up. While formal stretching may not be the recommended recipe, it's far crucial to warm up the muscle organizations and activate the frame in schooling for a run. This may be completed thru doing a little smooth leg swings to spark off the hips and wake up the encircling muscle tissues. You will need to maintain right now to a few component stationary and start gently swinging one leg at a time backward and forward some instances and in a circular motion out to the left or right. A few swings on each factor gets the muscle groups and joints activated and equipped to paintings. Activating the muscle organizations is crucial now not satisfactory to heat up the frame however additionally to make sure which you are awakening the more dormant joints and muscle tissue wanted for healthy strolling. A massive majority of humans spend maximum of their day sedentary at college or paintings. This can purpose our hips, quads, hamstrings, and one among a type muscle companies and joints to deactivate or emerge as dormant. If someone is then to pop up out in their chair for the day, slap on a few taking walks shoes, and take off, the frame does not have time to reactivate the dormant muscle groups and joints that would reason one-of-a-kind frame elements like your again muscle tissue to compensate main to harm or introduced ache. By spending only a few mins previous to strolling to set off your full frame, essentially waking it up from an afternoon of sitting, your frame may be extra prepared to keep you for your run with every muscle and joint doing the mission meant for it. This is simply one instance of why it is so critical to warmth up preceding to strolling, notwithstanding the fact that that doesn't imply a whole-on stretching session. The leg swing will however supply the muscular tissues a hint awaken stretch however preserve the danger of muscle weak point and decreased ordinary overall performance low.

Once you have completed a run, it's far important to commit 10-15 minutes to a short sit back out and stretch. Finishing a run and right now jumping on your automobile to strain home or hopping at the couch is not encouraged. During your run your muscle agencies will fill with lactic acid, that is the crucial aspect thing in ache. Lactic Acid is a chemical your frame produces to expose carbohydrates into strength, so famous it is a amazing element. However, after you complete your run lactic acid will continue to be on your muscle groups and is credited for the ache you feel in the days to conform with. Stretching is a fantastic way to increase blood drift through the muscular tissues and get rid of lactic acid and in the long run lower discomfort. However, it is crucial to pay attention to your body and do no longer overdo it. Depending at the quantity of try at some point of your run, it is vital to now not push your worn-out and weakened muscle groups too a long way. Immediately after a run it's miles endorsed to stretch out the legs, ft, and again very passively. Sometimes that can be as easy as genuinely doing a beforehand fold and letting your fingers maintain down. You need to feel this frequently on your hamstrings and decrease once more. It is a awesome manner to gently help the muscular tissues release the lactic acid while furthermore now not pushing the weakened muscle mass to a degree that could cause a pressure or tear.

To in reality see a difference in ordinary overall performance and popular mobility, your stretching need to move beyond in reality the earlier than and after. Integrating a plan into your every day recurring is assured to provide severa benefits to no longer super your overall performance on the identical time as walking, but everyday wellbeing and flexibility. There also are many unique techniques to stretch that we will cover in extra detail as we bypass. Dynamic Stretching is energetic movement where the joints and muscle tissue bypass through their entire sort of motion. This is the shape of stretching that we referred to earlier while specializing in earlier than the run. Whereas static stretching is keeping a stretch for some seconds close to its furthest factor and then, if appropriate, barely pushing past that aspect for an exceptional shorter duration of delivered stretch. This is just like the form of stretching after a run, besides we do now not need to push beyond the furthest factor after a more rigorous run to keep away from strains or tears inside the muscle fibers. There is likewise stretching referred to as Proprioceptive Neuromuscular Facilitation (PNF) stretching. This is wherein someone will settlement the targeted muscle businesses in quick at the same time as preserving the stretch. This shape of stretching no longer first-class will boom flexibility but additionally strengthens the muscular tissues. The following chapters will dive into the special styles of stretching more, but the bottom line is if you are inclined to put in a chunk more artwork each day, the advantages ultimately (truly) can be exponential.

Chapter 9: Dynamic Warm Up Stretching

Dynamic stretching is the usage of targeting energetic movement to loosen up the joints and muscle groups permitting them to prompt and increase your regular overall performance. Moving your joints via their entire variety of movement will help to prompt the joints and muscle mass and boom stability. By shifting through some easy motions, you can spark off your middle, hips, and leg muscle tissue. The incredible part of that is it most effective takes some short minutes and can be carried out quite a good deal everywhere. Here is a listing of numerous dynamic stretches alongside facet descriptions of a manner to perform them:

Leg Swings:

1.   How to do it: Hold onto a sturdy floor for stability, swing one leg earlier and backward, then transfer to the opposite leg. Aim for round 10-15 swings in step with leg.

2.   Benefits: Improves flexibility and mobility in the hip flexors and hamstrings.

3.   Muscle Groups: Engages the hip flexors, quadriceps, and middle muscle groups.

Walking Lunges:

1.   How to do it: Take a large leap forward, bending each knees to ninety ranges. Push off the front foot and trade legs while walking beforehand. Aim for 10-12 lunges on every leg.

2.   Benefits: Enhances hip flexibility and strengthens the quadriceps and glutes.

3.   Muscle Groups: Targets the quadriceps, glutes, and hamstrings.

High Knees:

1.   How to do it: Jog in area, bringing your knees as immoderate as you may. Aim for 20-30 seconds of non-stop high knees.

2.   Benefits: Improves decrease body coordination and cardiovascular staying power.

three.   Muscle Groups: Engages the hip flexors, quadriceps, and middle muscle mass.

Butt Kicks:

1. How to do it: Jog in place, bringing your heels up toward your glutes with each step. Aim for 20-30 seconds of non-stop butt kicks.

2. Benefits: Warms up the quadriceps and stretches the the the front of the thighs.

3. Muscle Groups: Targets the quadriceps and hip flexors.

Ankle Bounces:

1. How to do it: Stand on one leg, gently bouncing up and down on the ball of the foot. Switch legs and repeat for 10-15 bounces on every foot.

2. Benefits: Improves ankle stability and mobility.

3.   Muscle Groups: Engages the calf muscle groups and lets in with ankle flexibility.

Hip Circles:

1.   How to do it: Make round motions collectively with your hips, rotating clockwise and then counterclockwise for 10-15 repetitions every way.

2.   Benefits: Enhances hip mobility and flexibility.

3.   Muscle Groups: Targets the hip flexors, glutes, and internal thigh muscles.

Torso Twists:

1.   How to do it: Slowly twist your higher body to and fro even as

maintaining the decrease body robust. Aim for 10-15 twists on every issue.

2. Benefits: Warms up the center muscle tissue and will increase spinal mobility.

three. Muscle Groups: Engages the obliques, lower lower decrease back muscle businesses, and center stabilizers.

Arm Circles:

1. How to do it: Start with small circles and regularly growth the diameter. Do each ahead and backward circles for spherical 10-15 repetitions.

2. Benefits: Increases shoulder mobility and warms up the shoulder joints.

three.   Muscle Groups: Engages the deltoids, rotator cuff muscle mass, and better returned muscle tissues.

These are only a few of the vital aspect dynamic stretches that allow you to heat up and put together for your run. Each dynamic stretch gives precise benefits in terms of getting ready the frame for motion, enhancing flexibility, and concentrated on muscle corporations. You will see that numerous of these stretches goal the identical muscle and joint institution in tremendous approaches. Incorporating even some of those stretches into your heat-up routine can assist save you damage and optimize typical standard overall performance for the duration of physical interest. However, it's miles critical to take into account dynamic stretches must be performed in a controlled way and by no means forced into painful positions. The goal isn't always to move the joints and muscle corporations beyond a comfortable limit, but as an possibility you're definitely basically waking them up and allowing them to understand they will be approximately to go to art work. The moves should lightly put together the body for movement without causing strain. Adjust the intensity and period consistent with your health degree and normally make sure right shape whilst doing the ones physical activities.

Chapter 10: Static Stretches For Runners

Static stretching for runners facilitates enhance flexibility and can useful resource in preventing injuries with the aid of elongating the muscles and growing their style of motion. It is crucial to bear in mind that if you are stretching without delay after a run you want to pay interest very cautiously to your frame and maintain the stretches very passive. The muscle groups are worn-out from the exertion and if you push beyond the component of resistance, you run the chance of a tear. I have to recommend doing a little simple static stretches proper now following a run actually to hold the muscle tissue unfastened for the force domestic or brief bathe. Then, strive plopping down in the front of the TV with a yoga mat a bit later and supply the muscle businesses a more thorough stretch. Always preserve in thoughts that your body will inform you in which the bounds are, and it is important that you concentrate. Here is a list of static stretches for runners, collectively with the way to do them, the advantages, and the muscle corporations they purpose:

Quadriceps Stretch:

1.   How to do it: Stand on one leg, capture the ankle of the opportunity leg, and gently pull the heel in the course of the glutes. (You many need to maintain directly to a table sure object for balance)

2.   Benefits: Improves flexibility in the the front thigh muscle companies.

3.   Muscle Groups: Targets the quadriceps.

Hamstring Stretch:

1.   How to do it: Sit at the ground with one leg straight away and the alternative foot in competition to the internal thigh. Lean in advance, reaching inside the direction of the ft of the prolonged leg.

2.   Benefits: Increases flexibility in the again of the thighs, glutes, and espresso decrease returned.

3.   Muscle Groups: Targets the hamstrings, glutes, and quadratus lumborum.

Calf Stretch:

1.   How to do it: Stand dealing with a wall, location your hands at the wall at

shoulder pinnacle, step one leg again, and press the heel into the floor, maintaining the decrease lower back leg straight away. Slightly lean in advance inside the route of the wall to increase the stretch.

2.   Benefits: Aids in stretching the calf muscle tissue.

3.   Muscle Groups: Targets the gastrocnemius and soleus muscle organizations within the calves.

Hip Flexor Stretch:

1.   How to do it: Kneel on one knee, preserving the possibility foot flat on the floor, and lightly push the hips in advance.

2.   Benefits: Helps in stretching the the front of the hip and the hip flexors.

three.   Muscle Groups: Targets the iliopsoas and rectus femoris.

IT Band Stretch:

1.   How to do it: Cross one leg over the alternative, then lean to the issue, some distance from the crossed leg, engaging in overhead.

2.   Benefits: Stretches the iliotibial band alongside the aspect of the leg.

3.   Muscle Groups: Targets the iliotibial band.

Adductor/Groin Stretch:

1.   How to do it: Sit on the floor, convey the soles of the feet collectively, and lightly press the knees inside the path of the ground.

2.   Benefits: Increases flexibility within the internal thigh muscle mass.

three.   Muscle Groups: Targets the adductor muscle groups within the groin.

Piriformis Stretch:

1.   How to do it: Lie in your back, circulate one ankle over the alternative knee, and gently pull the lower knee toward the chest.

2.   Benefits: Stretches the piriformis and permits alleviate tightness in the glutes.

3.   Muscle Groups: Targets the piriformis and glute muscle tissues.

Lower Back Stretch:

1.   How to do it: Lie on your all over again and pull each knees towards the chest, protecting them together together with your palms.

2.   Benefits: Relieves tension within the decrease again and promotes flexibility.

three.   Muscle Groups: Targets the quadratus lumborum and spinal erectors.

Performing the ones static stretches after a run, whilst the muscle corporations are warmness, can useful resource in reducing muscle anxiety. Gently, keep every stretch for 20-30 seconds and carry out on each components to maintain muscle balance and symmetry. If you need to cognizance on gaining more flexibility and alleviating submit run ache, these static stretches also are a first-rate desire for an active rest day. On an energetic relaxation day, in which the muscle groups are improving, settle inside the the the front of the tv or switch on your favourite track and stretch a hint bit deeper. This is the correct time to slowly take those stretches a bit farther pushing through a hint little bit of the resistance. However, you may even though need to warmness up a bit either with a few brief dynamic stretches or without a doubt something as easy as a beforehand fold, in that you bend on the waist and drop your chest within the route of your legs simply letting your arms swing a chunk. This will permit the muscles to warmness up a piece preceding to a deeper stretch, supporting to avoid pulling or tearing cold, stiff muscle tissues.

five

Proprioceptive Neuromuscular Facilitation (PNF) Stretching Techniques

Another fantastic choice for stretching at once after a run is utilising Proprioceptive Neuromuscular Facilitation stretching. Proprioceptive Neuromuscular Facilitation (PNF) stretching is an advanced shape of flexibleness education that objectives to decorate both energetic and passive variety of motion in muscular tissues. This approach consists of a aggregate of stretching and contracting muscle companies to beautify flexibility and energy. PNF techniques are normally implemented in scientific settings, rehabilitation, and sports activities sports schooling due to their effectiveness in growing flexibility and useful movement.

The beginning of PNF stretching can be traced lower lower back to the Nineteen Forties whilst Dr. Herman Kabat, a neurophysiologist, in conjunction with physical therapists Margaret Knott and Dorothy Voss, advanced this approach. Initially, PNF modified into used in the rehabilitation of sufferers with neurological conditions to beautify motor characteristic. It turn out to be primarily based completely on the precept of stimulating proprioceptors (sensory receptors in muscular tissues and tendons) to elicit neuromuscular responses that might enhance muscle general overall performance. (ipnfa.Org, 2022)

The number one requirements of PNF encompass stretching a muscle to its limit and then contracting it statically towards resistance. This contraction is belief to loosen up the muscle spindles, bearing in mind a deeper stretch. There are diverse PNF techniques, with the most commonplace being the Hold-Relax and Contract-Relax strategies. These include a mixture of passive stretching, isometric contractions, and relaxation to growth shape of movement and versatility. PNF stretching focuses extra on strengthening the muscle mass via stretching. PNF stretching is top notch for stabilization and strengthening muscular tissues in a greater managed and static country. The contraction also permits to increase flexibility and may on occasion reduce the ache or pain that incorporates stretching. PNF stretching can be useful for runners as it allows decorate flexibility, strengthens the muscles, and might aid in decreasing the hazard of damage. Here are some simple PNF stretches generally used by runners, in conjunction with commands on a manner to carry out them, the benefits, and the targeted muscle businesses:

Hamstring Stretch (Straight Leg Raise):

1. How to do it: Lie to your decrease again with one leg extended at once at the ground and the other leg raised. Loop a strap or belt throughout the foot of the raised leg. Gently pull the leg in the direction of your chest till you revel in a stretch within the hamstring. Push in competition to the strap or belt at the side of your foot for 5-10 seconds. Relax and pull the leg similarly into the stretch.

2. Benefits: Improves flexibility in the decrease back of the thighs. Reduces tightness, supporting to enhance walking stride and save you injuries.

3. Muscle Group: Targets the Hamstrings

Quadriceps Stretch (Contract-Relax):

1. How to do it: Stand up immediately, bending one leg backward and grabbing the foot/ankle in the back of you. Gently pull your foot closer to your glutes until you feel a stretch inside the front of your thigh. Push your foot in opposition on your hand on the equal time as resisting collectively along with your hand for 5-10 seconds. Relax and pull the foot in addition in the direction of the glutes.

2. Benefits: Enhances flexibility inside the the the front of the thigh. Helps improve stride duration and wellknown leg extension.

3. Muscle Group: Targets the quadriceps.

Calf Stretch (Gastrocnemius and Soleus):

1. How to do it: Stand going thru a wall, placing your palms closer to it at shoulder height. Extend one leg returned collectively collectively with your heel at the floor and the knee right now. Lean forward, retaining your returned heel on the ground till you enjoy a stretch inside the calf. Push in opposition to the wall collectively together together with your forefoot for five-10 seconds. Relax and lean into the stretch in addition.

2. Benefits: Improves ankle flexibility and decreasing calf tightness. Helps save you commonplace going for walks-related troubles like shin splints and Achilles tendinitis.

three. Muscle Group: Targets the gastrocnemius and soleus.

Hip Flexor Stretch:

1. How to do it: Kneel on one knee, with the alternative foot flat on the ground within the the front of you. Keeping your torso upright, lean forward barely until you sense a stretch in the the front of the hip. Push your hips forward and settlement your hip flexors for five-10 seconds. Relax and lean similarly into the stretch.

2. Benefits: Enhances hip mobility and reducing tightness. Aids in

enhancing stride period and ordinary hip movement in some unspecified time in the future of strolling.

three.   Muscle Group: Targets the hip flexors.

Wall Adductor/Groin Stretch:

1.   How to do it: Lay all the way down to your again and positioned your legs directly up the wall developing a ninety degree mind-set. Slowly slide the heels down the wall preserving the legs directly in a V-form, attractive the inner thigh muscular tissues. Contract your adductors for five-10 seconds. Relax and slide your heels down the wall similarly.

2.   Benefits: Strengthens and stretches the adductor muscular tissues.

three.   Muscle Groups: Targets the adductor muscular tissues within the groin.

Table Hamstring Stretch:

1.   How to do it: Find a strong table. While reputation, enlarge one leg and rest it on the desk at hip height, lightly press your heel towards the table and lean ahead, engaging your hamstring muscle corporations. Contract your hamstring for five-10 seconds. Relax and lean beforehand greater.

2.   Benefits: Aids in developing hamstring strength and versatility.

three.   Muscle Groups: Targets the hamstrings.

Performing the ones PNF stretches often can motive stepped forward flexibility, advanced kind of movement, and reduced muscle tightness, which can be all beneficial for runners, helping to beautify normal typical performance and decrease the risk of damage. Ensure that you exert a slight quantity of pressure with out sudden movements to experience the benefits. Hold each stretch for 20-30 seconds with 5-10 second contractions in some unspecified time in the future of. Avoid overexertion through shifting slowly proper into a deeper stretch after every contraction. You in no manner want to yank and forcefully pull your body deeper. These could be a high-quality detail to comprise on your energetic relaxation days. Setting aside even as little as 10 min to do the ones stretches to transport your body right into a deeper stretch the usage of this approach will no longer best help you maintain muscle balance and growth flexibility, however it's going to moreover beautify your walking typical overall performance.

6

Yoga for Runners

Yoga gives many blessings for runners, enhancing each their physical and intellectual well-being. Adding a yoga exercise on your regular regular is each exceptional incredible manner to preserve your muscle tissue and joints limber and active. Yoga is essentially the all-in-one stretch, as many sequences embody both dynamic and static poses which might be alleged to target the whole frame. Yoga poses attention on stretching and increasing muscle mass, tendons, and ligaments, which reduces muscle stiffness and improves sort of movement. The postures, also have interaction severa muscle agencies, assisting in normal frame strength, which enables better walking form, staying strength, and balance. As a runner stability is important mainly while running on choppy surfaces like trails and plenty of yoga poses require balancing and attractive your middle muscle mass, which are crucial for retaining balance and right posture even as walking. A more potent core can beautify on foot common performance and reduce the risk of lower once more pain.

Along with the bodily blessings to runners, yoga consists of respiratory physical games that focus on deep, controlled respiratory. Learning to modify respiration styles can gain runners with the beneficial aid of enhancing endurance. It can also help with managing respiration for the duration of extended-distance runs, preventing humidity, or race day/schooling run tension. Running is full of surprises and sudden conditions which could purpose strain and anxiety, having the exercise to respire through those situations and refocus your mind and frame may be the distinction among completing a race or calling it quits. Learning to understand and schooling meditation strategies sell rest and strain discount that you could take with you to your greater hard or daunting runs. Sometime our minds can come to be our very very own worst enemy on an extended training run or race day. We can convince ourselves we aren't suitable sufficient or that the ache we're feeling isn't surely worth it.

Having the equipment to refocus the ones bad thoughts, breathe through the pain, and push forward can all come from a foundational yoga exercise. At its roots, yoga encourages mindfulness and the improvement of a strong thoughts-body connection. This heightened recognition can help runners better understand their our bodies, manage ache, and improve intellectual attention on the equal time as the going receives tough.

Regular yoga exercising also can assist prevent injuries via strengthening the frame and addressing muscular imbalances. Additionally, it may beneficial aid in restoration thru selling blood flow, decreasing muscle pain, and increasing mobility.

Overall, the blessings of integrating yoga into your education plan are endless. Signing up for a yoga splendor more than one times steady with week in your energetic rest days is a notable way to begin, but in case you are not prepared to decide to a class or financially now not in a position, no problems. There are plenty of free, on-line movies on the internet to assist get your started out out. Many of which can be targeted in the direction of specific desires, like strolling. It is vital to find out a stability amongst strolling and yoga durations to obtain the incredible results. Even incorporating short yoga lessons after an much less complicated education run a few times consistent with week can considerably effect a runner's performance and common properly-being.

www.ingramcontent.com/pod-product-compliance
Lightning Source LLC
Chambersburg PA
CBHW051728020426
42333CB00014B/1204